THE SOBERING TRUTH

What You Don't Know
Can Kill You

THE SOBERING TRUTH

What You Don't Know
Can Kill You

Jeff Herten, M.D.

SECOND EDITION

© 2025 MILL STREET PRESS
SAN LUIS OBISPO, CA

THE SOBERING TRUTH
What You Don't Know Can Kill You

Copyright © 2025 by Dr. Jeff Herten

All rights reserved. No portion of this book may be reproduced, stored in a retrieval system, or transmitted in any form or by any means–electronic, mechanical, recording, scanning, or other–except for brief quotations in critical reviews or articles, without the prior written permission of the publisher.

Softcover ISBN 979-8-9926222-0-1

ePub ISBN 979-8-9926222-1-8

CONTENTS

Acknowledgments 7
Introduction 9
1   Realization 13
2   You're Different When You Drink 19
3   How Alcohol Makes You Drunk 23
4   My Life With the Bottle: Part 1 27
5   Death by Alcohol Poisoning 39
6   Death by Chronic Alcohol Poisoning 45
7   Teen Choices that Last a Lifetime 51
8   Alcohol and the Adolescent Brain 57
9   The Brainwashing of America 59
10   Alcohol and Your Health: The Great Hoax . . . 69
11   Alcohol and Cancer 71
12   How Does Alcohol Cause Cancer? 81
13   Alcohol and the Heart 85
14   Alcohol and Hypertension 89
15   Alcohol and Depression 91
16   Alcohol and Osteoporosis 93
17   Alcohol and the Immune System 97
18   Alcohol and Allergies 99
19   Alcohol and GERD 103
20   Alcohol and Peripheral Neuropathy 105
21   Alcohol and Insomnia 107
22   Alcoholic Encephalopathy 109

23	Alcoholic Hepatitis	113
24	Alcoholic Pancreatitis	117
25	Alcohol, Obesity & Diabetes	119
26	Cirrhosis	123
27	Lesser Known Health Problems Due to Alcohol	125
28	Fetal Alcohol Syndrome	129
29	My Life With the Bottle: Part 2	135
30	Sarah's Story—Guest Author	143
31	Allison's Story—Guest Author	155
32	Alcoholic and Addicted Doctors	161
33	Observations of a Highway Patrol Officer	169
34	Scott	175
35	I Have an Excuse	181
36	Reactive Drinking	185
37	Bud	189
38	Concealing the Problem	199
39	The Drunk in the Boardroom	207
40	Ernest Hemingway	211
41	Alcoholism and AA	215
42	Lessons from the Liberty Tattoo Clinic	219
43	Enabling	225
44	Alcoholism: Criteria	231
45	How I Got Sober	241
46	Informed Consent	247
	Works Cited	252
	Appendix One	253
	Appendix Two: The 12 Steps of Alcoholics Anonymous	257

ACKNOWLEDGEMENTS

This book needed to be written to explain to unwitting consumers that a universally consumed substance has many more negative aspects than positive. It was inspired by my own personal relationship with alcohol, with encouragement from Dr. Bud Beecher whose recovery resulted in many years of successful teaching at Cal Poly. It was brought to fruition through the editing skills of longtime friend, Jane Broshears. It is dedicated to the countless millions of men and women who have had successful and fulfilling lives in recovery.

THE SOBERING TRUTH

INTRODUCTION

Supernatural joy is in no way that kind of dissipation, relaxation, and license by which too many people try to forget their human dignity.
— MOTHER MARIE DES DOULEURS

Ethyl alcohol, a simple hydrocarbon, is the most addictive drug on the planet; not because it is the most pharmacologically addictive, though it may be, but because it is the most accessible, seductive, and legal drug available.

Why is it so addictive? Somewhere on the way to intoxication, there is a brief moment when we feel so good. It is a feeling of well-being and no worries produced by the dissolution of inhibitions that alcohol effects. It is by removing these inhibitions, these little anxieties that we tote, that alcohol works its magic. It is the feeling we seek when we've had a grueling day at the office and want to relax with a glass of wine. It is the emotionally at-ease state we desire when we enter a room full of intimidating people at a party and head directly for the bar. It is the invigoration we strive for when we are emotionally exhausted and need a boost. And it is the amusing, happy-go-lucky attitude that our friends enjoy in us after we've had that first beer.

Unfortunately, that special feeling is fleeting. As we continue to drink, it disappears, and intoxication replaces it. Having experienced the feeling, we keep drinking, hoping more alcohol will restore it. It doesn't. But we keep trying. And in the process, we develop a psychological and physical dependence, an addiction to this all-pervasive drug. Alcohol is the most destructive drug on the planet. It has killed more people, directly or indirectly, than anything else except war and plague. It is responsible for more human misery than any other drug, more homicides, spousal and child abuse, sexual assaults, traffic deaths, violent crimes, and diseases of abuse. Those whose first addiction is alcohol often also become habituated to methamphetamine, cocaine, heroin, and prescription painkillers.

If alcohol were introduced today as a new product, its legal sales would be fought vigorously. But it's not new. Alcohol is so much a part of our society that it seems downright un-American to oppose it. What would a baseball game be without a beer? How can we eat a choice top sirloin without a good Cabernet?

So we succumb to our history, peer pressure, and effective media and marketing mind control. And we accept it. And we drink it. And slowly and insidiously, we become addicted. Alcohol morphs us into an unfamiliar character:

- A comedian who's the life of the party until he gets ridiculous and pathetic
- A Romeo until he can't achieve an erection
- A fearless superhero until he becomes aggressive and belligerent

I grew up thinking that every family in America celebrated happy hour. Dad would come home after work and drink two stiff highballs. And on New Year's Day, friends would gather around the television for the Rose Parade and drink screwdrivers and Bloody Marys. For special occasions, there were gin fizzes and rum punches. Every occasion was built around or served as an excuse for consuming varying and increasing amounts of alcohol. It took me fifty-four years to come to my senses, to see alcohol as the mind-altering, addictive, health-destroying substance that it is.

So let me take you on my odyssey, the ever-narrowing maze of a deluded person who looked at life as a series of opportunities to celebrate anything and everything with a drink. Let me introduce you to some characters who shared my travels but fell victim to the effects of the drug long before I did. I will describe what it's like to die of alcohol poisoning in a one-night binge or from thirty years of hard drinking. You'll meet, among others, highly effective, successful, productive people who all have one terrible secret. They are drunk nearly every day, and they can't function without alcohol. These are the high-functioning alcoholics

INTRODUCTION

(HFAs), and they comprise a large proportion of our society.

Ten percent of men and 5 percent of women are hard-core alcoholics. Recent studies show that 30 percent of Americans are binge drinkers, in that they get drunk at least once a month. But there are no accurate statistics for HFAs because they are largely invisible in our culture, except to their wives, children, and secretaries. They are very uncommon drunks, but they are drunks just the same.

Allow me to present to you the scientific facts on the health hazards of alcohol, facts you've never heard or read before, facts the marketers of a multibillion-dollar industry don't want you to know. For example, regular alcohol intake increases the risk of developing cancer, osteoporosis, birth defects, allergies, and infections. The alcohol industry has kept the truth from public awareness, so you may be shocked and amazed at your lack of information. But after reading this book, you will know the truth about alcohol.

I need to tell this story because, after more than thirty years, I am free from:

- The uncontrollable need to drink
- The despair of waking up every morning and knowing I had lost again in the battle against this addiction
- The certain disaster that was waiting for me and is waiting for every alcoholic, as the ever-tightening downward spiral sucks us into helpless, hopeless abandonment of dignity, reason, and sanity to a two-carbon poison called ethanol.

If this narrative awakens a single person heading for the abyss; prevents one needless traffic death, one episode of spousal or child abuse, or one case of cancer; or restores the dignity and humanity of a solitary soul, it will have served its purpose.

THE SOBERING TRUTH

1

REALIZATION

As shadows lengthened across the valley, the early sunset brought bone-chilling cold to the desert. Even in winter, Death Valley is forbidding. It proved to be the perfect place for a reckoning.

I was tired. I had ridden fifty miles on my young horse, Tuggy, from Panamint Springs just west of Death Valley to the Saline Valley and back. It was New Year's Eve, and the party was in full swing. I had drunk five or six beers, and I was visiting with friends at a table in the big tent while the country western band was on a break.

Some kids were seated with the backs of their chairs against the far end of our table. They were wrestling and giggling, and their chairs kept banging into the table, jarring it. Glasses bounced with the vibration, spilling wine and champagne. The kids looked over, recognized the nuisance they were creating, and kept right on wrestling. *Where are their parents? These kids don't belong at an adult New Year's Eve party.*

After another hard lurch of the table, I'd had enough. I walked over to the kids and firmly grabbed the nearest by the back of his neck. Startled, he squirmed away, rising from the chair.

Tightening my grip, I forced him down into his chair and growled at him. "You kids need to find another place to play." As I loosened my grasp, he twisted away, and he was gone.

It was a dull party, and I left after a couple more beers. As I departed, fellow rider and longtime friend, Ellen, approached me.

"Do you know Tommy Holden?"

"Who's that?"

"A little boy. He says you grabbed him by the neck and hurt him. His neck is bruised."

"What?"

"He said some drunk grabbed him, and he pointed you out. I told his mom I'd look into it."

The words hit me like a slap in the face. "Listen, Ellen, those kids were deliberately banging our table. I just sat him down. He squirmed away from me, so maybe the skin got pinched under his jacket."

"I saw his neck, Jeff. It's bruised."

"Ellen, I didn't mean to hurt the kid. I was only trying to get his attention."

"I'll talk to his mom and try to explain."

I went to bed, but I didn't sleep. I couldn't believe I hurt the boy. It seemed as if I'd barely touched him. I wasn't drunk. The seven or eight beers I drank were spread over five or six hours. Yet the fact remained that he was hurt. And I had done it. I was sick with guilt and humiliation.

What had he said? "Some drunk" grabbed him.

I knew there were times when alcohol made me angry and surly, but I had never hurt a child before. I saw myself through the eyes of that young boy, a big, mean drunk who grabbed him and slammed him into the chair. That was me. In the morning, before the drive home, I had to meet with the boy's mother. All the denials in the world couldn't change the fact that his neck was bruised. I apologized feebly and prayed the encounter would end. I didn't try to defend myself. My actions were indefensible. I listened to an outraged mother and just looked at the ground. Mercifully, it finally did end.

Alone on the long drive home, I experienced the most severe depression I have ever known. I was sick at heart, and I could understand why someone who felt this disconsolate could end his life. The psychological pain I experienced was close to unbearable. In the silence of the truck, I carefully dissected all the circumstances that had brought me to the flash point. I was physically exhausted from riding one hundred and fifty miles in the last four days. I had been taking ibuprofen for knee pain that resulted from the riding, and I had been, as usual, drinking. I had read that chronic ibuprofen use could cause severe depression, which certainly could have been a factor. I was sure the exhaustion contributed to it. But, in the depths of my soul, I knew the real cause was the alcohol and the losing battle I had been waging to control it.

It became painfully clear. I was miserable, and alcohol was the cause. I didn't want to drink. Gone was the exhilaration that followed the second beer. Gone was the jovial person who enjoyed a drink or two with friends. I became a sullen, surly, and depressed person who hated how alcohol made him feel.

I had tried numerous times to quit. I had failed every time.

I felt so weak and flawed. I couldn't respect this person I had become. Now I had let my addiction turn me into a physically assaultive person. I had hurt a child.

I had become a common drunk. I fantasized a video of me unsteady, slurring my words, and bullying a child. The realization was repugnant. In desperation, I vowed that I'd somehow finally find a way to quit. I'd free myself from this curse that threatened to ruin my life.

But denial is a formidable force. Back at home, in my comfortable environment, I rationalized I merely needed more control over my drinking. With my strong willpower and iron discipline, I could become a social drinker. I could drink like everyone else.

I first limited my drinking to Friday and Saturday, only two beers each night, for two weeks. Then there was a midweek dinner with friends.

What the heck? A couple of beers wouldn't hurt.

But it was more than a couple. The craving returned with a vengeance. I had failed again.

Ashamed and fresh with the memory of my New Year's Day humiliation, I knew I had lost control of my drinking yet again. Moreover, I had the frightening awareness that many alcoholics experience. I may never be able to overcome it. That fear caused despair beyond anything I have ever known. I found myself on my knees, praying in desperation to a God I hoped was there. It was different this time. I surrendered my will and ego to that power and asked Him to do what I could not. For the first time, I gave up and allowed Him to take control.

In what can only be described as a miracle of grace, my prayer was answered. A power beyond my own was there and still is. It was Ash

Wednesday, the beginning of Lent. It seemed most appropriate that I would give up that which was keeping me from a deeper awareness of God, that which was verging on destroying my life. Thus began my sober life.

Four months later, I experienced a second miracle, a confirmation of the first, something that could never have occurred if I were still drinking. My sobriety made it possible for some remarkable veterinarians to save the life of a horse I dearly love, my magnificent bay gelding, Famus.

My wife, Debby, and I were part of a group riding the historic Pony Express Trail from Missouri to California. A month into the ride, on a blistering hot day in Wyoming, Famus' intestines shut down. The resultant colic caused him unbearable pain. He stretched as if to pee and pawed the ground, frantically trying to ease his suffering. The vets attending the ride treated him for over six hours with no improvement. They made it very clear that, if I couldn't get him more aggressive care, the poisons fermenting in his stagnant gut would destroy his kidneys within hours. The only option was a four-hour trailer ride to the veterinary school at Colorado State. It was an hour before midnight. In my drinking days, I would have consumed four or five beers by then and been unfit to drive. Even though exhausted from an eight-hour ride in the heat, I was sober and committed to saving this very special friend.

I made the four-hour drive through the Wyoming night, towing my beloved Famus to the vets at Fort Collins. Miraculously, they saved him. Two days later, I returned to the ride, leaving behind a convalescing but healthy horse. I carried with me the memory of the long night of prayer to the same power that gave me the strength to quit drinking and the resultant calm certainty that Famus would survive.

On the return drive northward, I thanked God that he had given me the presence of mind and sobriety to save Famus. As my eyes filled with tears of gratitude, I received a clear message that I could express my thanks in tangible form by sharing my story with others.

In a nearly four-decade-long struggle, I had finally learned the truth about alcohol. I am free, no longer a slave to alcohol. It no longer owns or controls me. My newfound freedom has provided me undeniable peace and contentment. I look back on those dark days of addiction and marvel at what a blessing it is to be sober. Yet I see people who are struggling as I was and want to help them experience the joy of real freedom from addiction.

It is time for me to share my story with others, deluded as I was, suffering as I was, and denying as I was. I made a promise that day on the drive north to Casper. It has taken me over eight years, but I have kept it. Every time I grew tired or discouraged, I'd look out in the pasture to see that gorgeous bay gelding, remember that miracle, and get writing again.

Getting sober was just the first step. Since then, I have gained remarkable insights into the insidious and pervasive disease that alcohol has become for so many individuals and for our society as a whole. It has been an awakening.

This book will relate my story and the experiences of others who became addicted to alcohol. In every case, alcohol fulfilled a need. Perhaps you will see a similarity to your use of alcohol. You will become aware that alcohol is often used unsuccessfully as a coping mechanism.

In addition to its highly addictive nature, alcohol produces a multitude of negative side effects. So, when and if you do finally realize that alcohol is not helping you cope, it's often too late. You're already hooked. Another negative consequence of looking for an external fix is that you never dig deep enough to find the source of power within that can handle anything. Discovering that strength can be a life-altering experience rewarded by peace and self-satisfaction.

Does sobriety seem like an unattainable goal? It's not. The wonderful news is that it is never too late to change. Freedom from alcoholism is possible. It requires knowledge, understanding, and resolve. This book is designed to provide the first two and help you or your loved one find the last.

Let's get started. This is my prayer:

That my success in overcoming my alcohol addiction might help you to acknowledge and overcome yours, or it might help a loved one who needs to know the truth about his problem and find the willingness to change.

THE SOBERING TRUTH

2

YOU'RE DIFFERENT WHEN YOU DRINK

"First the man he takes the drink. And then the drink it takes the man."
— TOM RUSSELL

You might have inferred from the last chapter that I was a serious alcoholic. I wasn't. I never got sloppy drunk. I never got sick, never fell down, and rarely felt bad the next day. I never drank during the day. I'd never dream of drinking at lunch and going back to work. I never drank myself senseless or went on a binge. I was a well-respected physician in my community and taught on the faculty of the medical school. I never clouded my judgment with alcohol ... until the workday was over.

Then I'd stop off at the local liquor store and pick up a six-pack of one of my favorite beers. I'd crack one just after I turned up the country lane on which I live, and I had it down before I reached my driveway just over two miles up the road. I enjoyed the cold, refreshing taste, but the speed with which I drank it reveals I was doing it for one reason, how it made me feel.

I'd drink a second beer as I fed the horses, and that warm euphoria would ooze through me. Inwardly, there would be a long sigh as all the cares of the day faded away. But the feeling would be fleeting, and I tried to regain it with another beer at dinner and sometimes another after that. If you phoned after dinner, you might hear a little slurring at the edge of my speech. I became self-conscious about it, and I'd rarely call anyone or answer the phone after dinner.

I functioned at a very high level most of the time. I didn't consume that much, but I drank almost every day. I was addicted to alcohol, and it ruled my life. I refer to myself as a high-functioning alcoholic (HFA). There are millions of us. You may be one. So what's the harm? People like me are not a menace to society. We just have a few drinks after work to unwind. There's no harm there.

At first, maybe there isn't. My dad was like that. Every night, he came home and had two double scotches, bourbons, or vodka and tonics. The liquor depended on whatever phase he and Mom were in. It seemed innocent enough. But at the dinner table, more and more often, he would become argumentative. He'd single someone out, usually my sister, Julie, and pick a fight with her. It didn't matter about what. And he would pursue it until he had insulted and ridiculed her in front of the rest of the family.

Sober, my dad wasn't like that. He was one of the sweetest, most loving, and sentimental men on earth. So how could he so readily demean his daughter? He couldn't. It wasn't him. It was the alcohol.

This scene is repeated thirty million times at dinner tables all over America. Kids stare at their dinner plates, afraid to look up and become the target. In many households, it's not an argument. It's a brawl. Some poor kid is slapped, punched, or slammed against a wall. God forbid, the baby is a little colicky and begins to cry. A drinking dad may not have the patience for that. So he shakes that crying baby or slaps that whining child. It isn't really who they are. It is who they are with two gin and tonics or four beers in them. But the injured and frightened child doesn't know that. All he knows is that his home is a place of senseless fear and pain.

Many angry and abusive parents are not your textbook alcoholics. A large proportion of them are like me. They function well in society, and they have successful careers. They are well-respected members of the community. But they still drink too much too often, causing problems for their families and themselves. They are HFAs, like me. But they are alcoholics just the same.

Is there such a thing as harmless drinking? Am I completely opposed to alcohol? I know I am totally opposed to alcohol for me and others like me. I have an addictive personality. It took me fifty-four years to come to the awareness that I cannot drink, even a little bit, without it becoming a problem. And for a significant proportion of drinkers, I think that is true. Are there people who can just have a glass of wine at night and not have it get them eventually into trouble? There are, but I believe they are far fewer than we expect. If they drink wine, what are they drinking for? Is it for the nose or the wonderful aroma of fermented grapes that can take on such amazing subtlety and complexity? Perhaps, but in order to taste and compare a number of wines, one has to consume a significant amount of alcohol. Certainly, some can handle it without being drawn into the downward spiral that is addiction, but a substantial percentage cannot. It just fuels the growing problem.

It is a very individual situation, and only that particular person knows, if he is truly honest with himself, if he drinks for taste and aroma or if he drinks for the effect the alcohol has on his brain. If it is the latter, then he has the potential to get into trouble.

THE SOBERING TRUTH

3

HOW ALCOHOL MAKES YOU DRUNK

Alcohol is unusual in that it is absorbed right through the mucosa (the lining of your mouth, esophagus, and stomach). It is such a small molecule that it doesn't have to be broken down by any digestive enzymes, so it passes directly through the wall of any portion of the gut. This is in distinct contrast to most foods containing the three major energy sources: carbohydrates, proteins, and fats. Most of these are large, complex molecules that must be broken down into smaller molecular fragments by stomach acid or digestive enzymes in the mouth or small intestine to be absorbed. Absorption of alcohol begins immediately after the first swallow and continues until the last fragment is absorbed in the small intestine. Unlike many foods and most medications, alcohol is 100 percent absorbed into the bloodstream, and it is quickly and evenly distributed to all organs, muscles, fat, and, of course, the brain.

Because alcohol is so chemically simple, the body assimilates it very quickly. Its small size and simple structure allows it to pass readily through the membrane of every cell in the body. Alcohol functions as a two-carbon sugar, so it is considered to be in the carbohydrate family. It is metabolized preferentially over glucose in the liver and converted to a chemical called *acetaldehyde* at a fixed rate of one ounce per hour. Acetaldehyde is a toxic, cancer-causing chemical, and that toxicity is responsible for a large portion of the damage alcohol does to the body.

The higher the blood alcohol level is, the higher the acetaldehyde concentration also is. Alcohol is a cell poison. At high concentrations, it interferes with normal cell metabolism, and it is toxic to many cells in the body, including the liver, heart, and nervous system.

A small amount of alcohol is absorbed through the mucosae of the mouth, esophagus, and stomach. The majority is absorbed in the upper part of the small intestine. This portion of the small bowel is responsible for the absorption of many of the vitamins that are necessary for normal bodily function. Alcohol partially inhibits that absorption, causing alcoholics to be deficient in crucial vitamins. These vitamin deficiencies produce many of the long-term deleterious effects of alcoholism. Many alcoholics do not have the intake of vital nutrients essential for normal cell functions, especially the cells of the central nervous system.

Once absorbed, the alcohol is carried into small veins in the wall of the intestine, which coalesce into larger veins and eventually form the large portal vein that carries the ethanol and all other digested and absorbed nutrients to the liver to be processed. Everything that is ingested orally must pass through the liver before being distributed to the rest of the body. So the liver is the most vulnerable to the toxic effect of alcohol and all other poisons. The liver alters what it can of the alcohol, breaking it down to acetaldehyde, but it can handle only an ounce an hour, so the overflow enters the general circulation to intoxicate the rest of the tissues.

Alcohol is an equal opportunity intoxicant. It poisons all cells to the same degree. But some cells, like nerve tissue, are much more sensitive and prone to damage than others are. Fat is relatively insensitive to damage because alcohol is not very soluble in it. Fat does have a large reservoir of blood vessels, however, and the effect of dilution of a larger blood volume allows the ingestion of higher doses of alcohol with a relatively lower blood alcohol level. Nevertheless, all tissues are affected. Alcohol is soluble in the aqueous world of our tissues, so it passes readily into every cell.

Alcohol has the most notable effect on the nervous system. This system functions by an interchange, release, and reuptake of a number of chemical messages that are highly complex and not fully understood. When alcohol enters a nerve cell, it alters the amount of the chemical message the nerve cell releases, and it changes the reuptake of the chemicals that are critical for the cells to function normally. Very quickly, nerve cells develop a dependence on the presence of alcohol for the chemical message to be released.

The overall effect of alcohol is the suppression of neurotransmitter activity initially resulting in inhibition of control centers in the frontal lobe. Thus, in low concentrations, alcohol is a mild stimulant, and it may have a slight anti-anxiety effect as well.

The alcohol circulating in the blood is carried to the kidneys. Here, it inhibits a naturally occurring substance called *antidiuretic hormone* (ADH), producing a brisk *diuresis* (increase in urine production). Beer drinkers have to urinate a lot because alcohol is a diuretic. Chronic alcoholism can cause dehydration of all the cells in the body, a fact that makes drinking and exercising in hot weather dangerous for the unwary. Hot tubs can also be hazardous for acutely and chronically intoxicated people. Because they are already dehydrated with a low blood volume, alcoholics dehydrate further in the heat of the tub. If the blood volume gets critically low, blood pressure may plummet. There are more than a few accidental deaths every year due to intoxicated hot-tubbers.

Alcohol may cause the kidney to excrete more calcium due to increased urine production. The speeded-up flow of urine prevents the kidney tubules from reabsorbing calcium. Alcohol also increases urinary loss of calcium by altering levels of parathyroid hormone that are responsible for its conservation. Because of these effects, chronic alcohol intake leads to a long-term loss of bone density.

Acute intoxication causes muscle cell death because of the toxic effect of ethanol. Alcoholic myonecrosis may be mild, but, in severe cases, enough myoglobin (the large oxygen-carrying protein in muscle cells that is similar to hemoglobin) may be released from dying muscle cells to stain the urine a vin-rose color. The myoglobin can even plug *glomeruli* (millions of tiny little filter apparatuses) in the kidneys and produce kidney failure. Chronic alcoholism leads to muscle shrinkage or atrophy and weakness.

Because the heart is a muscle, it is vulnerable to the toxic effects of alcohol as well. Long-term exposure produces an alcoholic cardiomyopathy, which weakens the heart and can produce congestive heart failure.

As it circulates through the body, alcohol produces a mild dilation of blood vessels, especially in the skin. This produces the flushed face of the acutely intoxicated and may contribute to the large, dilated veins seen on the cheeks and nose of many drinkers. To be fair, many other factors contribute to the facial veins, such as heredity, sun, and diet, but there is little question that, if a person is predisposed to this problem, alcohol use will aggravate it.

The alcohol-caused dilation of blood vessels in the skin may result in a prompt and dramatic heat loss as the warm blood, reaching the surface, radiates heat into the surrounding environment. Acutely intoxicated people are at great risk of hypothermia in a cold environment because they are losing heat to the air, and alcohol decreases their sensitivity to the effects of the cold. This accounts for the death of many alcoholics from exposure each winter.

When considering the many short- and long-term effects of alcohol, two questions arise:
- Why isn't educating the public a higher priority for health-care professionals?
- Once people are educated, will they continue to drink? And if they do, why?

Hopefully, the information in this book will help to answer these and other questions. Perhaps it will convince you to rethink your present drinking habits or those of your friends and loved ones.

4

MY LIFE WITH THE BOTTLE: *PART I*

Beer is one of my oldest friends. My first recollection of drinking was sitting on the front lawn with my dad after he'd finished mowing the lawn and getting a sip of the Olympia beer he quaffed on a hot summer afternoon. The fizzy bubbles tickled my nose. The taste was bitter, but with a subtle hidden tingle. I learned to love that taste. When I started drinking beer in earnest in college and later, it never tasted the same or as good as it did on those hot summer Saturdays. I was eight years old. I never got more than a single sip, but special times with Dad became associated with drinking.

They were called "French 75s," named for the storied cannons of World War I. Made from champagne and brandy, poured in a tulip-stem glass, they were my first real taste of alcohol. I was about fifteen. We were at our neighbor's house for a Christmas open house. Jack McDougall decided the kids would be allowed to try one. We were each given our own glass of the sparkling elixir. I felt the bubbles all the way down my throat and up my nose, but I liked the taste. A half hour later, I had the most peculiar sensation. I felt warm all over. A gentle heat started at the top of my head and spread slowly down across my face, neck, torso, and out to the tips of my fingers. It proceeded all the way to the bottoms of my feet, which itched in an odd way. It felt very strange but good, like the world was smiling. Everything was okay. A little while later, I felt fuzzy. My vision was slightly blurred. I was momentarily frightened, but then it passed. I was experiencing the effect of alcohol for the first time.

There was a myth when I was in high school that two aspirin and a Coke would make you tipsy. I tried it on a youth group weekend retreat at Yosemite, trying to impress a young lady with how sophisticated and cool I was. Although it didn't work, I acted intoxicated anyway. She was not impressed. It's interesting now to reflect on how important and mature I was trying to feel by getting intoxicated. Sadly, I had already learned some lessons from my family life about the importance of altering my mood with alcohol to feel good.

My best friend in high school was a bright, sarcastic, and worldly boy named George Townes. We had been on a debate team together in Forensic League and were members of the same high school YMCA club. George had a wonderful sense of humor, and he was fun to be around. He also had a drinking problem. His parents were both in the motion picture business. Like my parents, they drank heavily and saw no problem with George drinking along with them. They were gone often, especially on weekends. George would help himself to their bourbon or scotch and take me for a ride in his Plymouth with the push-button transmission. There were some hair-raising rides on the narrow, winding roads of the Hollywood Hills, lurching around tight corners and screaming along straight stretches of Mulholland Drive at ninety miles an hour. It's a wonder we weren't killed, but the thought never entered my mind. I was just exhilarated. I did not drink then. I was a late bloomer socially and rather straight, but I did enjoy my crazy friend.

George went off to the University of Washington and continued his drinking unabated. In his freshman year, at a fraternity party, he drank himself almost unconscious. Stumbling out of the party, he slipped on some ice and struck his head on solid concrete. He was in a coma for just shy of a week. When he recovered, he couldn't remember his class schedule or how to drive to the campus. Eventually, it all came back, but it scared him into never drinking again. George is now an English professor at a major university, and he is completely sober.

Similarly, college almost killed me. I was seventeen years old, socially very immature and suddenly alone in a culture where alcohol was venerated, almost worshipped. It began the summer before my freshman year with fraternity rush parties, poolside gatherings at fabulous homes in Palos Verdes or dances in funky beer halls near campus. The prospective pledges were sure to be introduced to the big-name athletes of each house. And there was lots of beer. I was cautious about drinking more than a couple of glasses. I had never really been drunk, and I didn't want to create a negative impression, as drinking was still a mysterious and unexplored journey for me. I had watched my parents for years, so I knew how people acted when they drank. I had also observed my uncle, who was always sloppy drunk and rude at holiday family gatherings, but I hadn't had the experience firsthand, so I was very tentative. The fraternities were careful not to let the rush party drinking get too out of hand. The hard-core drinkers were warned about getting drunk and insulting the rushees. Instead, they paraded all their athletes, student leaders, and notable alumni by us during these parties. These were handsome, clean-cut guys in button-down shirts. But there was always the beer. And there was no question that we were expected to drink it. No one abstained at these functions. I don't remember a single person at any of these parties, male or female, who didn't drink.

I immediately joined a fraternity that was well stocked with all-American swimmers, golfers, and trackmen. My sister, a member of one of the better sororities on campus, considered it to be very cool. Sadly, I didn't pick the group of young men by any criteria other than the reputation they had around campus, and I didn't wait several semesters to really assess what was happening in the Greek system. I was young and insecure, and I wanted a social anchor in the very imposing university life I was beginning. So I pledged.

Several weeks after the end of rush, the house had a big party. A bus was hired to take a large group out to a small lake on the outskirts of the city. Several of the upperclassmen had driven down to Mexico to buy gallons of white lightning (99 percent ethanol). Placed in grape and lime Kool-Aid and poured into empty beer kegs, it became purple passion and green death. Members, pledges, and their dates filed onto the bus, and the party and drinking began immediately. I drove separately because my date was an old high school girlfriend who was just beginning her senior year and I had to pick her up at home.

We had a little trouble finding the venue. By the time we arrived, the party was in full swing. A band played on a large swath of grass along the shore. A few couples were dancing while many sat around the lawn, listened, and drank. I knew what was in the punch and warned my date not to drink too much. Many were uninformed or unwise. Several hours, a sunken canoe, a broken rope swing, and untold numbers of retches later, forty couples staggered back to the bus and headed for campus. When they arrived back at the fraternity, the sides of the bus were decorated with vomit including chunks of pineapple with faint green and purple streaks.

I drank several of the punches, but didn't feel drunk. My date, a little tipsy, snoozed on my arm as I drove home. Just as I reached the freeway, brilliant red lights appeared in my rearview mirror. A cold fear gripped me as a spotlight illuminated the interior of the car. I rolled down the window, and a highway patrolman shined a light in my face.

"May I see your driver's license?"

"Yes, sir. Is there a problem, officer?" I handed him my opened wallet.

"Please take it out."

I removed it and handed it to him.

"Did you know you had a taillight out?"

"No, sir. It's my dad's car, and I only drive it on weekends."

He handed the license back to me. "Were you at the party at the lake?"

"Yes, sir."

"Have you been drinking?"

"Yes, sir."

He studied me for a long minute. I was seventeen years old. Any drinking at my age was illegal, let alone driving under the influence.

"You better be going straight home, young man."

"Yes, sir." He turned and strode back to his patrol car as I wilted in a sigh of relief.

This was 1965. The no-tolerance policy for alcohol that exists now was years in the future. A kindly man took pity on a basically good kid and let him go. I wonder how different my life would have been had I been cited. A 502 (driving under the influence) on my record might have ruined my chances for medical school. I was definitely the recipient of a gift of grace that night. It's too bad I was too young to experience the awakening I did when Tommy Holden labeled me "some drunk" at that New Year's Eve party. But I couldn't imagine all the misery that alcohol would bring to friends and acquaintances and me. I had no insight, no point of reference other than my upbringing in a drinking family. No one prompted me to question if this was sane or healthy behavior. So rather than learn a lesson, I felt I'd had a very close call. I learned not to drive with burned-out taillights and use backstreets and out-of-the-way routes to get home when I had been drinking. Through the grace of God, I never have been stopped or cited for driving under the influence.

The next day, I bragged to my fraternity brothers about being stopped. I was typical of many young people, both then and now.

Boys, of course, are the worst. Part of it is the testosterone, which fuels aggressive behavior, coupled with a lack of maturity in adolescent boys. A fascinating recent study showed the male brain does not fully mature until the early-to mid-twenties, providing some explanation for the dangerous and irrational behavior of teenage boys (CDC Fact Book 2001–2002).

My college fraternity fostered institutionalized alcoholism. The Christmas party was a perfect example. After picking the name of a brother out of a hat, each fraternity member bought that person a gift, invariably booze. One of the upperclassmen, dressed up as Santa Claus, arrived at the party, already inebriated. Very few Santas made it through the Christmas party without passing out, throwing up, or both. At the party, Santa would pick a gift, read the tag, call the recipient up, and have him sit on Santa's knee while opening it. Then the recipient had to drink it. Most of the time, the gift was hard liquor. Tequila was particularly popular. Mescal was too, especially Cusano Rojo, a large square, yellow, liquid-filled bottle with a hideous, coiled, red worm at the bottom. The challenge was to take a big chug and swallow the worm.

My drinking skills made me somewhat of a legend one Christmas when I chugged a gallon of red wine. The cheap and popular Red Mountain came in gallon jugs. I chugged half of it, went outside, and stuck my finger down my throat. I vomited the first half and then came back to finish it off. I vomited most of the second half as well, but not enough to avoid a horrific headache the next day during my inorganic chemistry quiz.

Given the large amount of hard stuff that was consumed, it was a wonder that no one died of acute alcohol poisoning. It is very simple to kill yourself by drinking. If you consume alcohol faster than your body can metabolize it and you don't get sick and vomit before it reaches a toxic level in your bloodstream and brain, you can die. It happens several dozen times a year on college campuses.

Sometime late in my sophomore year, my girlfriend and I broke up. In a ritual observance of grief, I publicly drank myself unconscious. It was a night of open houses on fraternity and sorority row, and I carried a half-gallon of Spanada (a poor attempt to re-create sangria) with me as I accompanied friends to the other houses. I tripped over a privet hedge and fell down at some point in the evening. I barely made it back to my fraternity house before I passed out.

I awoke the next morning, lying fully clothed on my bed, covered with vomit in varying stages of drying. I remembered nothing of getting sick. I didn't know then that a common secondary cause of death in acute alcohol poisoning is aspiration pneumonia, a process where corrosive stomach acid and enzymes are inhaled or aspirated into the lungs of stuporous or comatose individuals. These potent chemicals literally digest lung tissue, producing large pockets of necrotic tissue and pus. There is no satisfactory treatment for aspiration pneumonia. If it isn't fatal, it often destroys large amounts of healthy lung tissue and leaves its victims respiratory cripples with diminished lung volumes and recurrent infections. Again, my guardian angel somehow turned my head to the side so the vomit decorated my pillow instead of filling my bronchi. I had no idea how lucky I had been until years later. I studied aspiration pneumonia in medical school. When I was an intern, I treated two cases that were fatal. I had a long-term reminder of the incident, however. Some of the vomit had splattered on my shoes, a pair of oxblood Florsheim Imperial wingtips that my dad had bought me when I left for college. The acid vomitus had digested away the shiny veneer and left dull spots that would never take a shine again. I had those shoes for twenty years, the dull spots reminding me of my alcoholic brush with death.

MY LIFE WITH THE BOTTLE: PART I

It was both a blessing and a curse that I tolerated alcohol well. I am a moderately tall guy, and I was a little chunky, which was helpful because alcohol is evenly distributed in all tissues. Even though it is not very soluble in fat, adipose tissue is richly supplied with blood vessels, effectively diluting the alcohol and lowering the blood alcohol level and thus the effective dose. Big people, fat or not, can drink a great deal more, with less effect, than their small, thin counterparts can. But, in my case, there was more to it than that. I could match a friend who was the same size and body fat beer for beer and not act as drunk. I was just as drunk as he was, but something about my nervous system allowed me to function better with the same blood alcohol level. I could hold my liquor, and I was proud of that fact.

I functioned well after considerable alcohol intake, driving in a perfectly acceptable manner. When I had a great deal to drink, I would see double. That could make driving difficult. No problem! I found that, by closing one eye, I had monocular vision again and drove merrily and relatively straight down the road. This was the 1960s, and the police and highway patrol were not as vigilant as they are today. The real menace of drunk drivers was not as well understood or publicized in those days. Many of my college peers and I got away with it.

Another of my college drinking exploits occurred in a high-class bar and restaurant a few blocks from campus frequented by alumni, staff, and, occasionally, undergraduates. Behind the bar, neatly arranged in wooden holders, were long glass beakers that measured eighteen or thirty-six inches, the fabled half-yard and yard of ale popularized by our cultural, political, and alcoholic ancestors, the Brits. There were periodic contests to see who could chug a yard (three pints) of ale the fastest, and anyone could challenge the record at any time. A decent time for a yard was five seconds while most average beer drinkers might put it down in nine or ten seconds and be pleased. I had the questionable fortune of having the ability to open my throat and literally pour down the beer while also possessing a rather large stomach volume. When I graduated from college, I held the record of 2.9 seconds for a yard, a dubious honor. Thirty-five years later, I wish my academic accomplishments had been as outstanding.

Additionally, in the 1960s, the medical and psychiatric community knew the concept of the addictive personality, but it wasn't well known to the general public. If it were, perhaps I would have recognized the signs in myself. Besides, I was no different from 80 percent of the guys in my fraternity. These were my peers, and they all drank hard. I desperately wanted to be one of them. I didn't know anyone who abstained from alcohol. If I had, I would have thought they were nerds. I drank no more than the majority of my fraternity brothers and a lot less than some could. I didn't realize that we were all alcoholics-in-training. Sadly, most of us succeeded as HFAs, and a tragic few were terminal drunks.

In my junior year, a fellow student asked me to tutor him in philosophy. I was a decent student, getting by more on intelligence than study habits, having been seduced by all the distractions of college life. The son of a famous actor, he was wealthier than most of our peers were, and he was a very big man on campus. I was flattered to be asked.

We agreed to meet the night before the exam and cram. He picked me up, and we drove to his parents' opulent home in Brentwood. We began to study. By eleven o'clock, it was obvious we could never cover the material in time for the exam.

He pulled out several small yellow pills and handed me one. "This will help keep us alert to finish the job."

I didn't ask what it was, but I'm sure it was amphetamine, a potent stimulant and performance enhancer. We studied all through the night. The mental focus that the drug produced was quite remarkable. Philosophy had never been this interesting before.

When I wrote the exam the next day, I filled two blue books, and I could have filled more. I earned the highest grade in the class. My new friend got a B, and he was very pleased. I was amazed at the effect of this little yellow pill on my intellectual performance. It was a pharmacological epiphany.

Several postgraduate dental students still frequented the fraternity, occasionally for meals or a social event. In a casual conversation over a bridge game one evening, one of them intimated that most of the dental students took uppers to study. Could he get me some?

Yes, indeed.

My addiction to amphetamines began as simply as that.

I was involved in a great many student activities in college. Then a poor manager of time and a natural procrastinator, it was easy to put my studies on the back burner. I did go to class most of the time, but I did only a portion of the considerable reading that my classes required. It was easy to put off studying until the night before the exam, knowing I had a wonder pill that would allow me to cram three months of studying into an all-nighter and perform extremely well on the exam.

The last year-and-a-half of college, I used speed to study. The drug of choice was called Eskatrol, a prescription diet pill containing dexamphetamine sulfate, combined with a very mild tranquilizer to mitigate the shakiness and anxiety side effect of the upper. It was amazing stuff, producing six to eight hours of intense concentration and total recall. By graduation from college, I couldn't study without it.

On a warm spring afternoon at the end of my senior year, I used up two more of my nine lives. I was in emotional turmoil. I was elated because I had just received my acceptance to medical school, but I was greatly disturbed because the housemother of the sorority where I worked serving meals, a dear friend, had suffered a massive stroke. I was hosting a mixer between the senior men's honor service organization and a similar women's organization from the nearby Catholic university at my off-campus apartment. The party was in full swing, and the beer was flowing freely. The club members were all well oiled and pretty rowdy when Rudy, the apartment manager, arrived to investigate the commotion. I saw him coming down the drive and worked my way across the patio to intercept him, but I was too late. Unaware who he was, one of the members had thrown a cup of beer at the intruder.

Rudy stomped down the drive. I probably should have pursued him and tried to assuage his anger, but I was drunk and having fun. I figured he'd get over it.

I could apologize for my friends tomorrow.

I was at the hors d'oeuvres table when I sensed everyone turning toward the drive. There was Rudy, at the edge of the patio, holding a small pistol in the face of his tormenter. I was just drunk enough to have no fear.

Rudy would never shoot anyone. He's just saving his pride, frightening this rude drunk.

I moved unsteadily across the patio and stepped between them. Now the gun was in my face, but I was too drunk to be frightened. I apologized for my intoxicated friend and hardly took note of the blue steel barrel waving in front of my nose. Rudy made a good show of it, insisting I get out of the way so he could teach that *cabron* a lesson. Maybe he wouldn't shoot, but he was angry, the gun was loaded, and anything could happen when alcohol and firearms are involved. It was well known around the complex that Rudy had a drinking problem, so how did I know he wasn't drunk enough to do something stupid? I didn't, but, luckily, even drunk, I made the right call. After listening to my apologies for what seemed like an eternity, but was probably only a minute or two, he put the gun back in his coat pocket and walked down the drive.

When the mixer was over, I performed a cursory cleanup and decided to head downtown to the Pantry for dinner. I enlisted a friend, and we hopped into my 1957 Volkswagen bug. Miraculously, we both put on our seat belts.

I had not consumed any beer for an hour or more, but I was still feeling the half-dozen glasses I'd had at the party. I drove onto the freeway and got up to speed, moving over to the left for the transition road that would head north into the city. I was chatting with my friend when a car full of very attractive young ladies passed us on the right. Stan and I were very interested and attentive, and the girls were clearly enjoying the high-speed encounter. I beeped my squeaky little horn. As I did, I looked up to see the concrete railing of the tight turn of the transition road. With the distraction, I hadn't been paying attention, and I had failed to brake at the approach of the turn. I looked down to see seventy miles per hour registering on the speedometer. As I looked up, the only object in my vision was a large yellow sign with the word "SLOW" and an arrow curving to the left.

Even the quick reflexes of a twenty-year-old could not slow the Beetle quickly enough to handle the tight curve. I braked hard and steered left, but the car skidded to the right. Sliding across the lane, I saw the concrete rail looming ahead. I corrected back to the right, and the car responded by skidding to the left. The railing on the other side loomed up. I steered back to the right. The rear end of the car whipped around, and now I found myself in a four-wheel drift back the other way. I tried to correct yet again, but the torque was too much, and the car flipped. Everything seemed to be in slow motion inside the vehicle. I felt my door pop open and books and odd papers rained down and flew back again as we continued to roll. I counted two revolutions and then a slam as the chassis came to rest against the right side railing. Stan and I were hanging upside down, held in by the seat belts. Both doors had popped open. Without restraints, we would have certainly been ejected and crushed by the rolling vehicle.

The adrenaline produced by the crash and fear of being caught created an urgency and a sobriety that saved us. Stan and I unfastened our belts, fell to the ceiling (now floor), and climbed out. The front bonnet had popped open, and the spare tire was wobbling down the ramp. The engine was still running. We quickly rolled the Beetle back on its legs and climbed back in. The roof had been crushed down about a foot so the sprung doors no longer closed, but protruded above the roof, like the wings of a butterfly. We both held our respective door shut, and I steered with my right hand while Stan shifted with his left, driving around the transition road, down the off-ramp, and into the parking lot of the Pantry. We parked in a space that was out of view from the ramp or the street. At the time, it seemed like an exciting adventure, but, looking back, we were beyond lucky.

After this episode, my guardian angel applied for a transfer. By a miracle of good fortune, we weren't caught. I was just twenty years old, underage for drinking. Even though the standard for intoxication was higher (0.10 percent), my blood alcohol level almost certainly exceeded that at the time of the accident. I somehow managed to cheat death and avoid the societal penalties of my very poor judgment one more time.

I graduated from college a month later. Along with many of my classmates, I had developed a serious alcohol problem. I only drank on the weekends, but consistently to moderate intoxication. Alcohol was the constant companion at all social occasions, and it was used to celebrate the highs of life and mourn the lows. In the social environment of my college, alcohol was pervasive, and there were established rituals for experiencing both elation and sorrow, all of which involved getting drunk. Sadly, I never questioned the rationale.

Was the alcohol to heighten the joy? Salve the grief? Obscure the pain? Erase the memory?

It did none of those things, but it had become a strongly conditioned response to a wide variety of emotions.

PARENTS SUE FRATERNITY AFTER SON DIES AT PARTY

The parents of a University of Washington student who died in a fall at the Pi Kappa Phi house are suing the fraternity, saying he was encouraged to drink during a party game.

In the lawsuit filed this week in King County Superior Court, Don and Janice Jensen said that the May 2002 death of their nineteen-year-old son, Brett, followed a game called "Century Club" in which participants are supposed to drink a shot of beer every minute for 100 minutes.[1]

---

[1] *If the shot glass were an ounce-and-a-half, the participants would absorb nine ounces of alcohol in that period and have a blood alcohol level of 0.25 percent at the end of the game. If the shot glass were two ounces, twelve ounces would be consumed, resulting in a blood alcohol level of 0.35 percent.*

5

DEATH BY ALCOHOL POISONING

One minute, he was alive, talking about a mountain bike trip and plans for the holidays. Ninety minutes later, he was dead. Two fine young men killed themselves with alcohol in our town last year. One lived out by the state park where we ride our horses. Every time we trailer out there, I read a banner stretched on a fence along the road, "We miss you, Randy!"

And I mourn. Randy was a junior in high school. He and his buddy cut school and went to a friend's house to do some serious drinking. Incredibly, the friend's parents were home part of the time and knew (or should have known) what was going on. They had stolen a half-gallon of whiskey from one of their parents' liquor cabinet. They began to drink.

The drink of choice for killing oneself with alcohol is hard liquor simply because it has a much higher concentration of alcohol than beer or wine does. The alcohol builds up in the bloodstream faster, causing deadly poisoning before the side effects prevent or reduce the intake. It is possible to kill yourself with beer, but the lower concentration (6 percent) requires the consumption of much larger quantities. Before a fatal blood alcohol level is reached, the beer drinker may mercifully vomit or pass out. The same is true of wine, which, at 10 to 12 percent alcohol, requires the drinker to consume a larger quantity than hard liquor.

So when you are matching your friend drink for drink, guzzling several ounces of straight whiskey each time, you need to remember one critical fact. You can drink and absorb alcohol much faster than your liver and other tissues can metabolize and get rid of it, so the level is constantly rising. If your blood alcohol level reaches 0.4 percent before you pass out, vomit, or some-body stops you, you may just die. Randy did.

There is a dynamic process going on when you consume alcohol: consumption, absorption, and elimination. Alcohol is absorbed rather quickly and at almost 100 percent efficiency, so consumption is roughly equal to absorption. Elimination is variable, but within a relatively narrow range. The novice drinker can metabolize one to one-and-a-half ounces of alcohol per hour. A veteran drinker, whose liver has had repeated exposures to alcohol and is more efficient, may be able to metabolize half again that much, but there is a limit to how fast alcohol can be cleared from the body. That upper limit may approach two ounces per hour. The blood alcohol level depends on how fast the alcohol is consumed and how strong it is.

When large amounts of highly concentrated alcohol are consumed quickly, the normal stages of drunkenness are passed through, but very rapidly because the drug is being consumed and absorbed at such a high rate. And as a high school junior, you're not an everyday drinker, so your liver is not habituated. It doesn't metabolize the alcohol efficiently. Your friend is the same height, but weighs fifteen pounds more, mostly fat. Because alcohol is evenly distributed in tissues, he can drink 15 percent more than you can for each stage of intoxication.

At 0.1 percent blood alcohol level,[2] you are pleasantly buzzed. You feel lighthearted and happy. You're talkative and funny. All your worries seem trivial, and you have a warm glow. Your lips might feel a little thick, and your balance might not be perfect, but you could probably pass a field sobriety test. You would fail a blood or urine alcohol test and a breathalyzer because the legal limit for alcohol is 0.08 percent. You are feeling good.

At 0.2 percent blood alcohol level[3] as a rookie, you are feeling very drunk. Your speech is slurred, and your walk is quite unsteady. You may see double. You are not as mellow as you were, and you become loud and

---

[2] *Allowing for elimination of an ounce-and-a-half an hour, that is an accumulation of four ounces of alcohol or eight ounces of whiskey.*

[3] *This is a net surplus of eight ounces of alcohol or sixteen ounces of whiskey.*

DEATH BY ACUTE ALCOHOL POISONING

obnoxious as liquor dissolves normal social restraint. Males may still be able to get an erection, but it probably won't be a great one. And there might be real difficulty having an orgasm. You're just plain drunk.

Veteran drinkers may function surprisingly well at 0.2 per-cent. Their livers have increased enzymes for breaking down the alcohol, and both nerves and muscles have learned to adapt to higher levels of ethanol while still functioning adequately. Many high functioning alcoholics (HFAs) live their entire waking lives with a blood alcohol level of 0.2 percent. They drive, work, close big business deals, get pregnant, have kids, and, in time, can't function without it.

A friend of my parents, Jack McDougall, became enormously successful drinking a fifth of bourbon every working day and more on weekends. The boardrooms of the Fortune 500 companies are well stocked with HFAs who can and do function remarkably well with blood alcohol levels of nearly 0.2 percent. It's a given that they will have two drinks during a power lunch with prospective clients, pour a drink from their sideboard in the afternoon when they clinch the deal, stop at a bar across the street from the office before they leave for home, and have a couple of double highballs before dinner. It would stagger the imagination to know what proportion of high-level business executives are also HFAs.

After twelve ounces of alcohol,[4] the blood alcohol level climbs to 0.3 percent, and the staggering drunk falls down. Alcohol affects the higher centers of the brain first, that is, the cerebral thinking, reasoning, remembering, and emoting part of the brain. At increased blood levels, the midportion of the brain, the cerebellum, is affected, impairing balance and coordination. At yet higher levels of alcohol, the lower centers of the brain are affected as well. These are in the brain stem, which is in charge of consciousness, blood pressure, respiration, and temperature regulation.

When the blood alcohol level reaches 0.3 percent, most people pass out. If they are lucky enough to be in a temperate environment, a knowledgeable and caring soul may turn their head to the side to prevent them from choking on or aspirating their vomit. If they are unlucky and pass out alone in the cold, they could suffer hypothermia or freeze

---

[4] *This is a net gain of twenty-four ounces of whiskey.*

to death, as alcohol impairs temperature control and dilates capillaries close to the surface of the skin. They quickly lose their core heat to the surrounding cold and suffer hypothermia. Although my emergency room work occurred in a temperate climate zone, it was common to see drunks brought in comatose with body temperatures in the low nineties, a moderate degree of hypothermia. In severe hypothermia, core temperatures in the low eighties, cardiac arrhythmias occur and may lead to death.

Unconscious, the drunk may vomit, plugging his airway. Worse, the vomit may be aspirated or sucked into his lungs.

In a coma, the drunk may be insensitive to the damaging effect of hard surfaces on soft tissues resting upon them. A conscious or sleeping person shifts position when pressure on an area of skin becomes uncomfortable. A passed-out drunk does not. The result is pressure sores on the skin and occasional massive areas of necrosis or dead muscle and subcutaneous tissue.

After a net surplus of sixteen ounces of alcohol,[5] a blood alcohol level of 0.4 percent is reached, and death may follow. I say "may" because, with some veteran alcoholics, it may take a bit more. I was an intern at LA County-USC Medical Center during a severe flu epidemic. A reorganization of medical admitting had created an overdose ward, exclusively for doses to take the pressure off the overcrowding of the hospital with flu cases. Along with another intern, I was selected to staff the dose ward. One night, I admitted a comatose drunk named Billy, whom the staff knew well. I worked him up, started an IV, and drew some blood. He was stable and quiet in the corner of the admitting room when my attention turned to a new patient, a famous actor who had some heroin at a party that was much more potent than he anticipated. He was comatose and in respiratory arrest. By the time I had stabilized our celebrity, I looked over to see that Billy was gone. He had disconnected his IV and left without saying good-bye. Then the lab called with his blood alcohol level. It was 0.45 percent. We all just shook our heads. Billy set the record for blood alcohol level during my tenure on the overdose

---

[5] *This is thirty-two ounces of whiskey.*

ward. Just then, the phone rang from the ER. They were sending up a red blanket. The elevator doors opened, and beneath the red sheet was a comatose Billy. Apparently, he had passed out again on the front steps of the hospital. When security found him, he was not breathing. After a little CPR, an endotracheal tube, an ambu bag, and another IV, Billy was mine again. I was able to bring him back, but alcohol finally killed him several months later on another intern's watch.

Randy and his friend shared a half-gallon of whiskey. That's sixty-four ounces of liquor (thirty-two ounces of alcohol), and it killed him. He drank it so fast that he was able to reach 0.4 percent before he passed out, he got sick, or someone stopped him. When he finally did pass out, the alcohol level was so high that it stopped his breathing. Without oxygen, a heart already weakened by high alcohol levels cannot last long, perhaps a minute or two. Then it stops. And tragically, no one recognized what had happened in time to help. So the world lost another young person to alcohol and another bright and promising future that would not be. There was another devastated family, memorial service warning friends about binge drinking, and another obituary chronicling the life of a nice guy, promising student, and gifted athlete. And there was another sign on a fence, a memorial to a moment of bad judgment.

THE SOBERING TRUTH

6

DEATH BY CHRONIC ALCOHOL POISONING

Bruce Anderson was gazing at death as he stared up at me with terror in his eyes. His lids were drawn back, and the globes almost bulged out of their sockets. The whites of his eyes were the color of a crook-necked squash, jaundiced from the bilirubin (a yellow pigmented breakdown product of hemoglobin) in his bloodstream that a failing liver could not metabolize and remove.

Bruce was in hard restraints, heavy leather hand and ankle cuffs strapped to the frame of the bed so he couldn't flail about or pull out the tubes and IVs that were keeping him alive. A tube used to irrigate his stomach with ice water protruded from one of Bruce's nostrils. The tube was taped to the noseguard of a football helmet strapped to his head. He shook violently from delirium tremens (DTs), the chill of the ice water that was being flushed down the tube, and shock, having lost a third of his blood volume to gastrointestinal bleeding.

Bruce, an alcoholic in the end stages of liver failure, was bleeding from esophageal varices (varicose veins bulging into the esophagus caused by a scarred liver). It was his first bleed. There was a fifty-fifty chance it would be his last.

His beard was caked with clotted blood, his hair was matted, and his arms were covered with large purple bruises.

How did this happen to him?

One word.

Alcohol.

Bruce was thirty-nine years old. He began drinking in college with the seemingly harmless drinking games and bacchanalian rites of fraternity life. He graduated in engineering and then took a job as a technical sales representative for a medical device company. His work included dining potential customers. The two-scotch-and-water lunches and dinners on the company expense account were gradually preceded by a couple beers in the bar and a snifter of brandy and a cigar after dessert. Bruce made many sales. He was a good talker, even while drunk, and clients liked his humor and friendly manner. He was a HFA.

Bruce met and married a flight attendant, Jeannie. They were perfect together. She drank gin and tonics and became very sexy when she drank. They had an elegant townhouse in Marina del Rey and a small sailboat. Life was rosy, but short-lived.

It lasted eighteen months. Jeannie was two weeks late returning from a three-day trip. When she returned, it was to tell Bruce that she had fallen in love over gin and tonics with a pilot named Carl, and she was leaving. Bruce went on a bender. He missed work for a week. When he came back, irony and sarcasm had replaced the humor and friendliness. The two-scotch-and-water lunches became three-martini lunches. If he did return to work after lunch, he just shuffled papers on his desk. His sales fell off. His bitter sarcasm put off clients, and they grew tired of hearing how Jeannie had ruined his life. After three months in a self-destructive decline, Bruce was fired. He went on another bender and ended up in the county hospital detox unit. He was assigned a social worker, given a referral to a rehabilitation program, and sent home.

Bruce lost his townhouse and moved in with his brother. On his budget, he could no longer afford scotch so he drank cheap vodka. He found a job as a janitor in an office building downtown, but they let him go after repeated absences. His brother finally threw him out, and he went to live with his widowed diabetic mother. When she died, he found himself on the street. Bruce had made the transition from an HFA to a common drunk.

It took eleven years for the alcohol to ruin his liver. Little by little, high concentrations of alcohol killed liver cells. Fibrous tissue replaced them. Gradually, the beautifully complex liver was turned into a rock-hard mass of scar tissue, and Bruce developed cirrhosis.

Understanding the process that produces liver cirrhosis and all of the many medical problems that result requires knowledge of basic liver structure and function. The liver is a large (three-pound) organ that sits under the right diaphragm. Its jobs are legion. It receives all the incoming nutrients from the gut through a special set of veins called the portal system. Digested food is absorbed through the intestinal wall into small veins that travel to the liver. Here, the nutrients are metabolized by liver cells into usable proteins, fats, and carbohydrates. These then enter the general circulation for the body to use. The liver also detoxifies any hazardous substances or drugs that may be absorbed from the intestine. It is like a huge manufacturing and recycling center. It recycles the vital blood-carrying protein hemoglobin by accepting a by-product called bilirubin and altering it to produce the substance bile, which flows through ducts to the gall bladder where it is excreted back into the gut periodically to help digest fats. Finally, a network of immune cells in the liver is responsible for gobbling up foreign proteins, bacteria, and parasites in the blood that might be attacking the body.

When alcohol is absorbed through the gut wall, it travels to the liver where it damages hepatocytes (liver cells), producing varying degrees of inflammation termed *alcoholic hepatitis*. Hepatocytes are actually killed. In the resultant cleanup effort, they may regenerate, but the complicated connections to the incoming portal veins, bile ducts, and nutrient arteries are often disrupted. If severe enough, fibrosis or scarring occurs, and the complex architecture of this miraculous organ may be altered. With repeated episodes of alcoholic hepatitis, the scarring gradually narrows the incoming or portal veins. At some point, when the scarring is severe, the liver cannot adequately process the incoming portal blood from the intestine, and the blood backs up. The scarred liver produces a tourniquet effect on the portal veins. The resultant increased pressure in these veins causes them to bulge, and they may rupture when stretched to the extreme. The internal varices (varicose veins) thus created line the gut, including the esophagus, stomach, bowel, and rectum. Internal hemorrhoidal as well as esophageal varicose veins are the result of this high pressure in the portal system, a condition known as *portal hypertension*.

The massively dilated veins that line the esophagus are the most prone to bleed. Sharp-edged foods like potato chips or a fishbone might scratch the mucosal lining over one of these varices, or they might tear from the violent vomiting of acute alcohol intoxication. The instant these veins rupture, at least a quart of blood under pressure fills the stomach. Some is digested into melena (black, tarry ooze) that smells like death itself. Most is vomited as bright red blood.

Varices are thin-walled. Unlike arteries, they have little or no muscle in their walls. As a result, when shock sets in, there is no compensatory spasm of the muscular wall of the varices to stop the bleeding. They just bleed until there is no more blood in them. Not uncommonly, GI bleeders that are due to cirrhosis and varices exsanguinate (bleed out). Fatal shock and cardiac arrest quickly follow.

Bruce was bleeding out. When he arrived in my emergency medicine admitting ward as a red blanket, his pulse was rapid and thready, his blood pressure almost nonexistent. He had a large gauge tube cut down into the vein in his forearm, which had been placed in the emergency room before he was shipped upstairs. He had already been given two liters of Ringer's lactate and two units of untyped, uncrossed whole blood. There was no time to type the blood. He would have died without it.

My job was to pass the Sengstaken-Blakemore tube. It was huge, but, with KY jelly in his nostril and some luck, I got it down. It had a doughnut-like balloon just in front of the stomach end, and a small tube that ran along the sidewall of the larger tube could inflate it. I quickly filled the balloon with mercury, used for its weight. Once the balloon was inflated, I drew back on the tube, trying to make a seal around the cardio-esophageal junction, the neck of the esophagus as it enters the stomach. This is where esophageal varices most commonly bleed. Hopefully, this would compress the varices and stop the bleeding. It stopped for a while, and we were able to stabilize Bruce's blood pressure. With the acute emergency over, I was able to complete my physical exam.

Bruce was a textbook case on the physical findings of end-stage liver disease due to alcoholism. He was jaundiced from the failing liver. The bilirubin could not be processed by the failing liver, so it backed up in the blood and stained all the tissues of the body, including his skin and eyeballs. Because his liver could not manufacture bile to digest the fat in his diet, his stool was a whitish clay color. His skin was covered with large, red bumps called *spider hemangiomas* (small arteries that grow into the skin because of an excessive amount of estrogen in the blood). The adrenal gland produces estrogen, and the liver breaks it down. Without a functioning liver, Bruce's body had excess estrogen, also responsible for Bruce's large breasts and shrunken, almost absent testicles. So much for the myth that alcohol increases your libido. Bruce hadn't had an erection in five years.

He shivered from the shock of blood loss and the ice water lavaging his stomach. There was a coarser shake as well, perhaps the first sign of impending DTs. And there was yet a third movement, a slower, rhythmic cadence as his feet and hands patted the mattress. Large amounts of ammonia in Bruce's blood produced this liver flap. A normal by-product of metabolism, especially of proteins, ammonia is usually broken down and detoxified by the liver. Bruce's liver was no longer able to detoxify anything.

Bruce had a protuberant belly, caused in part by his enlarged, rock-hard liver and massive accumulation of fluid in the abdominal cavity. The same congestion and back pressure that created the portal hypertension also caused the liver to weep fluid (ascites), and his belly was full of it.

I was charting my findings after finishing my exam when the bottom dropped out. Bruce's blood pressure plummeted. Sensing impending doom, he began to thrash and writhe uncontrollably.

A death struggle can be a terrifying event to witness for the first time. Our inner primitive animal fights, often with superhuman strength and violence, to survive. So it was with Bruce. I watched, riveted, as every muscle fought against the restraints, bowing the steel rails of the bed to which they were anchored. Struggling to sit up as far as his bonds would allow, he growled a guttural sound, an utterance of anguish and fear. His fingers grasped for anything and clung with a death grip to the sheets and railing. His eyes, tightly shut with effort, suddenly opened and looked directly into mine. The look was of desperation and fear. Death hovered at the foot of his bed, and he was powerless to drive it away. Then the connection was lost, his eyes closed again, and he was abandoned to the mindless animalistic struggle. I turned the IV line wide open and hung another unit of uncrossed blood. The return from the nasogastric tube was pure blood. I tightened the tension on the tube, but, as I did, his pulse disappeared, his bulging yellow eyes rolled back in his head, the thrashing ceased, and his yellow skin turned blue. An hour later, after CPR, fluids, blood, and intracardiac epinephrine, Bruce got his wish. He had finally killed himself.

In the intern's sleeping room, I looked at myself in the mirror. Exhaustion was in my eyes. My face was spattered with dried blood. Bloody fingerprints were on my shirt where Bruce had tried, in his final agony, to get my attention, to somehow convey the terror he was feeling. And to swear that he could now finally quit.

7

TEEN CHOICES THAT LAST A LIFETIME

Every story in this chapter is true. Alcohol irretrievably altered every one of the lives involved. Alcohol caused a lapse in judgment, common sense, and motor skills resulting in consequences that would last a lifetime.

* * * * *

The voice on the phone was sobbing. "Mike, I'm pregnant. What are we going to do?"

You're numb. You can't believe what you just heard. The night it happened is a blurry memory. There was a party. Holly had been flirting with you all semester. That night, she was coming on big-time. You both had more than a few beers. The next thing you knew she was leading you downstairs. Unprepared, you had no condoms.

What are you going to tell your parents...her parents?

After one phone call, your life is changed forever. There's no more free time or hanging with your friends. You need to support and care for a baby 24/7. You're going to have to work at a minimum wage job after school until graduation. You can forget about going away to college. It will take you twice as long to finish, if you ever do. Your whole life changed in one wasted moment.

* * * * *

You thought Ty was going too fast, but, what the hell, it was a fun ride! There are shrieks from the backseat. Someone laughs as he throws a couple of empties out the window. The curve is too sharp, and Ty can't hold it. The car careens onto the right shoulder. Ty swings the wheel left, and the car spins into the oncoming headlights.

The lights drive straight into your door, the passenger side. There is an explosion of glass and a sickening crunching of metal. An instant later, there is another explosion and the smell of burning rubber. The crumbling frame pushes you toward Ty, and the hood of the oncoming car folds up in front of you. There are muffled screams from the backseat. There is grinding, scraping, and screaming. Then there is nothing.

Ty's door is sprung, and you both climb out around the air bags. There is sobbing from the backseat.

"Oh my God! My face."

There is a huge laceration across Cody's forehead, shaped like a trapdoor. Something sharp had ripped back a huge piece of skin. Jagged and ugly, it is sitting on top of his head. Blood is everywhere. Patrick isn't moving.

There are screams from the other vehicle. Smoke is pouring from the crumbled engine compartment. You run to the window. A woman is sobbing uncontrollably, rocking back and forth, cradling a man's head in her lap. Blood is pouring from his nose and eyes. He will die in her arms.

For you and Ty, the nightmare isn't over. It's just beginning. Vehicular manslaughter, DUI, and minor in possession, the list seems endless, and the sentence will be even longer. But it can't compare to the knowledge that your carelessness cost someone his life. Your whole life changed in one wasted moment.

* * *

You've just left Dave's after a few beers. You're heading home, driving cautiously to avoid being pulled over. You try not to drink and drive, but you had no other ride home. Somebody's tailgating you, flashing his brights for you to speed up. You pull up at a signal. A pickup with two guys in it pulls up beside you. The guy in the passenger seat gives you a dirty look, mouths "f____ you," and gives you the finger.

You are pissed off. You're trying to drive cautiously. These guys are giving you grief, so you return the gesture. Before you know what's happening, they both jump out of their truck with baseball bats. Your window is broken in an instant. You can't get away quick enough. They drag you out of your car. They hit you repeatedly with the bats. White-hot pain sears your head, back, and arms. You are down, covering your head. Now they are kicking you, stomping you with their heavy boots. Then everything goes dark.

You awake in the county hospital. Your head is throbbing, and it feels bigger than a watermelon. Your left arm is in a cast. Your nose is running briskly, dripping on your massively swollen upper lip. The drainage from your nose is cerebrospinal fluid leaking from a crack in the base of your fractured skull. The healing of the torn covering of the brain will put you at risk for seizures. You will need to take an anti-seizure medication, and you will not be able to drive for two years. You are lucky to be alive. Your whole life changed in one wasted moment.

You awoke that morning feeling a bit strange, a little achy. Halfway through algebra, you started feeling waves of chills alternated with fever so you skipped volleyball practice after school and went straight home. By the time you arrived home, you were feeling horrible. Every muscle in your body hurt, you had a splitting headache, and you were burning up. Your mother tried to make you drink fluids, but you just lay still in bed and didn't move. Everything hurt.

The pain and blisters in your vagina began on the second day. There was a burning, as though a torch had been placed up inside. Urinating was agony. You had to get into a lukewarm bath to void. Even then, it was painful.

After two days, you weren't better. Your mother took you to the doctor. It didn't take long to make a diagnosis. After one look at your vulva, the doctor said in an apologetic tone, "Sarah, this is Herpes simplex, type 2. This is a primary outbreak."

You were in shock. *How could that be?*

There is only one boy, Tom, and he always used a condom. Then you remembered that night after the basketball game. You had been drinking with some friends, and Zack was sitting by you. He was cute and sexy, and you got very drunk. You may have passed out, but couldn't remember. You were pretty sure you had sex.

Now this. What does it mean?

For the rest of your life, you will have recurrent painful outbreaks of blisters in your vagina, sometimes from sex, sometimes from stress, and sometimes from periods. You'll be contagious, even when you don't have blisters, to anyone with whom you have sex. And if you get pregnant, you may transmit the infection to your new baby if delivering while broken out. In order to prevent the infection from causing severe brain damage to your newborn baby, a C-section may be required. You will experience a lifetime of pain and embarrassment. After one wasted moment, your life was changed forever.

* * *

His parents were in the waiting room. Someone would have to tell them. You would be that someone. You don't need to give them the gory details; the bullet entered beneath the left eye, went through the maxillary sinus at an upward angle, entered the skull through the floor, tore through the meninges, and sliced into the base of the brain. You don't need to include that it compressed half the cerebral hemisphere against the skull as it exited, explosively ripping a three-inch piece of bone and skin off as it exited three inches behind the right ear.

It didn't matter now that his friend was just playing after they shared half a fifth of his parents' whiskey. It didn't matter that he thought the gun wasn't loaded. All they need to know is that he died instantly. After a bright flash, he was gone with no pain or suffering. There was nothing that could have been done once the gun was fired. But it won't be easy.

He was their only child, and he was nine years old. After one wasted moment, a life was ended.

* * *

Have you ever held a belief that was so strong that you never doubted it? And then, one day, you awoke to the realization that you had been completely wrong?

Maybe you had a friend you confided in and trusted, but found out she was sharing all your secrets with others. Maybe it was an unfaithful lover. Maybe it was a fact you learned in school that you thought was as solid as the law of gravity. Then, one day, you realized you had been mistaken all along.

Alcohol is like that. Everyone does it, and it feels so good. It adds to the enjoyment of friends and occasions. But not everyone can drink occasionally and moderately.

Don't start. What seems like so much fun at first can lead to untold misery. Suicide is the third-leading cause of death in teens (*Morbidity and Mortality Weekly Report* 2004, 471). In males, it is on the rise (*Morbidity and Mortality Weekly Report* 2005, 377). Many are alcoholics on the fast track to hopelessness and helplessness. Depression that is so prevalent in teens is compounded by the depression of alcohol. Remember that one wasted moment can change your whole life.

THE SOBERING TRUTH

8

ALCOHOL AND THE ADOLESCENT BRAIN

As if alcohol wasn't a serious issue at any age, it is doubly problematic for adolescents.

First, an immature brain will not mature fully in the constant presence of alcohol. Recent studies suggest that the human male brain does not fully mature until 25 years of age, the female until 23. Alcohol inhibits the synthesis of cholesterol in the brain that is necessary for the construction of nerve cell walls. Alcohol inhibits the brain's development toward maturity. A chronic alcoholic who began drinking at 12 continues to possess the intellectual and emotional maturity of a 12 year old well into his 20s and 30s unless he stops drinking.

Second, alcohol profoundly affects the pre-frontal cortex, that area in the brain that is responsible for impulse control, judgment, integrity, inhibition, and decision-making. That explains the dangerous behaviors, DUIs, STDs, sexual predation, unplanned pregnancies, and the progression to even more dangerous drugs seen in the adolescent population.

If we are to stem the tide, we need to educate children and adolescents in a way that they can appreciate the danger of alcohol use in spite of the pressure from the media, advertisers, and their peers. We also need to inform enabling adults and parents of the consequences of alcohol consumption at any age, but for certain in this most vulnerable segment of our society.

THE SOBERING TRUTH

9

THE BRAINWASHING OF AMERICA

The handsome young cowboy flirted with the young ladies at the boarding barn. He sipped a beer and groomed his sleek chestnut quarter horse before putting him back in the stall. A small knot of horsewomen gathered at the wash rack. They smiled, giggled, and blushed at his simple attentions. Tall, lean, friendly, and a good horseman, everyone at the barn liked the young man. A new student at Cal Poly, he was majoring in agricultural science, and he had a bright future. He paused to visit with coeds and sipped another beer. Then he was in his truck and on his way home. He never made it.

Driving out of town, he was going too fast for the curve and rolled his truck. Without a seat belt, he was ejected from the truck, and was airborne at fifty miles an hour. His head slammed into a brick wall at the entrance to a housing tract just beyond the curve. It nearly exploded from the impact. Mercifully, he was dead at the scene. Dead at twenty years of age. His blood alcohol level was 0.15 percent. The sudden loss stunned everyone at the horse unit.

·····

She was blonde and beautiful, and it was her twenty-first birthday. Cristal King promised her mother that she would not drive. After a night of celebration, she accepted a ride home from a twenty-three-year-old young man who had a prior DUI and was driving on a suspended driver's license. He was trying to impress her with the power and handling of his convertible sports car, but he misjudged the curve on the off-ramp, slamming the passenger side of the car into the retaining wall. The lovely young life in the seat beside him was instantly snuffed out. An only child, the pride of her loving and hardworking parents, was dead, her spectacular smile gone forever. The drunk driver didn't kill one person that night. He killed three. Her parents are dead emotionally, and they may never recover.

I remember the haunted face of Cristal's mother at the trial. Robbed of her only child, she wanted harsh punishment for the driver. His blood alcohol level was 0.10 percent, hardly enough to impair his driving ability, but certainly enough to impair his judgment. Convicted of involuntary manslaughter and sentenced to prison, his life will never be the same. A banner hangs on the retaining wall where she died, reading, "A Cristal clear reminder. Don't drink and drive." Her mother places bouquets of fresh flowers in a vase at the base of the wall in an attempt to keep her memory alive.

Two high school chums swigged a six-pack on a warm spring evening and decided to drive into town. The driver misjudged a curve, and the vehicle slammed into a huge oak tree at the road's edge. The passenger died. The driver suffered massive chest injuries, but survived to carry the physical and emotional scars of that night all his life. And incredibly, there were letters to the editor of the local paper the following week, stating the oak tree was a hazard and really needed to be removed.

A young mother was driving her two children to a soccer game. On the main street coming into town, a drunk young man passing on a two-lane road hit her head-on. One of the children was killed. The other spent a month in the hospital and months in rehabilitation. The drunk driver was unscathed physically, but will see the faces of those children and the grief-crazed, tear-stained face of the mother for the rest of his life.

Two young men with a twelve-pack of beer were out joyriding in a rural part of the county. The driver missed a curve, ran off the road, hit a power pole, and broke a fifteen-thousand volt wire, which dangled just outside the door where the car came to rest. The driver may have recognized the danger if he were sober, but he certainly didn't while he was drunk. He struggled out of the car and brushed the wire. He was instantly electrocuted. He was the oldest of three brothers, bright and handsome, captain of the football team, and headed to UC-Davis the next fall. His parents, brothers, and classmates were numb with shock.

An unsuspecting motorist was driving into town on Highway 1, slowing to fifty-five as he approached the first set of signals on the west side. Suddenly, a man walking beside the highway ran into his lane of traffic. The driver didn't even have time to hit the brakes. The pedestrian was dead on impact. The papers speculated the dead man, a student at Cal Poly, had committed suicide. But he was doing well in school, and his friends said he was not depressed. Two weeks later, a one-paragraph article reported that his blood alcohol level was 0.34 percent.

He shouldn't have been able to stand up, let alone walk. Where were his friends? Who let him leave the party that drunk? Was he really trying to kill himself? We'll never know. The only certainties are his death and the shocking impact on the motorist who hit him.

I live in a county with a population of 283,000. The local papers reflect the small-town feeling by featuring county news in the front-page headlines. Articles on traffic deaths keep me constantly aware of the tragedies that alcohol has created for so many. Every year, at least two of our high school students die in alcohol-related accidents. I often know their families. The whole community mourns.

I feel a great sadness whenever I read about another needless death. I visualize the devastated parents, shocked friends, and guilt-ridden driver. And the scenario plays out over and over again. Only the actors are different.

I also experience anger. When is our society going to recognize the devastating effects of alcohol on our youth? How will we stop this hemorrhaging of the lifeblood of our society, these beautiful young people who have a momentary, alcohol-induced loss of judgment?

The advertising industry and news media aren't behind us. They have brainwashed three generations of young people with the sexiness of liquor. It begins with kids in junior high and high school. All major sports events, the extreme sports, and popular television shows run beer commercials. And they are clever, sexy, and funny.

There are the extraordinarily attractive bikini-clad babes surrounding the guy who is drinking the right beer. Overt as well as subliminal, these messages suggest that the right choice in beer will guarantee getting the girl, being cool with your friends, or enhancing your snowboarding skills. For this pubescent audience, the importance of belonging to a peer group is paramount. Advertisers understand peer identification and effectively use it to enlist beer drinkers.

For the older age group, there are male-bonding scenes like watching the big game with the boys, made all the more poignant with the right beer. For the health conscious, there is the beer brewer sifting hops through his hand, ever so seriously explaining that beer is a natural food and emphasizing the importance of its freshness, which is why his company has breweries in every major city in the country.

For the patriotic, there's the magnificent beer wagon being pulled by the strongest, most beautiful draft horses imaginable. How can you not admire that? They have become cultural icons. Yet what are they promoting?

Is there something disingenuous about a beer manufacturer promoting responsible drinking? Is that an oxymoron? Now it's important to designate a driver, so everybody else in the group can drink more freely, consume more, and have a guilt-free drunk.

For the thirtysomething, upwardly mobile set, the delivery system for America's drug of choice is different. It is wine. It is incredible how the wine industry has grown in the last two decades. The association of sophistication with wine knowledge and appreciation has been one of the great marketing coups of the wine industry. Thirty years ago, the wine shelf in your local liquor store had one aisle of jug wines and a section of screw-top Tokays and ports for the itinerant wino crowd. Now, half the space in large liquor stores is devoted to thirty different wine varieties from fifty different wineries. Wine-tasting classes and wine clubs have developed in every small community, and better homes have temperature- and humidity-controlled wine cellars. What a remarkable advertising and promotional success!

Years ago, I was one of them. I swirled, swished, and sniffed the wine of the week with the like-minded folks. And we talked about legs, nose, and body, and we waxed poetic about the aromas.

"There's a subtle hint of clove here."

"Do you detect a bit of mint?"

"This wine has vegetable overtones."

And we took copious notes and stored them away in our files. I can't deny that I enjoyed those evenings and I learned a lot about wines and winemaking. But I also can't deny that I have seen many of those wine club friends drunk a good portion of the time at those meetings and formal wine dinners. Are we deluding ourselves? Is wine education just an excuse, a rationalization for getting drunk? For many, it is exactly that. If you disagree, answer one question. If it's the aroma, color, body, and subtle tastes that are really important, why not take the alcohol out? Nonalcoholic wines are available but unpopular. Wine drinkers want the alcohol. That's why they are drinking.

It was a brilliant coup for the wine industry when medical scientists published that one glass of red wine is good for the heart. What is often overlooked is that the study states "a glass," which is six or eight ounces of wine with dinner. I'm sure it is good for the heart. But people who drink only one glass of wine with dinner are as rare as smokers who smoke only one cigarette a day. For the HFAs of the world whose delivery system of choice is wine, that medical study legitimized their addiction.

In another remarkable advertising bonanza, the medical community published that moderate alcohol intake raises high-density lipoproteins

(HDLs), the good fraction of cholesterol. But studies demonstrating that moderate alcohol consumption also increases one's risk of developing a number of cancers, including breast cancer, aren't made available to the public. The powerful alcohol industry filters the information.

Public relations and advertising firms have created a grand illusion about the wonder of drinking liquor. Be observant of the ads on television, billboards around town, or displays at liquor stores and supermarkets. Notice how stacks of cases of beer are strategically placed where they intercept the most foot traffic. Observe the labels on the cartons celebrating whatever season we are in because every season is a season to drink.

Ironically, public opinion has swung so adamantly against cigarette smoking and the tobacco industry, but we still embrace fantasies about alcohol. Do you remember the old commercial for cigarettes produced during and after World War II? The star of the World Series is shown on a billboard, endorsing a brand of cigarette and claiming it improved "his wind." The rugged Western star offers that his brand of smoke improves his appetite. And people bought it. In view of our present knowledge, these advertisements are ludicrous. Given the deleterious health facts of drinking alcohol, so are advertisements about liquor. We have simply traded one poison for another. But the general public remains uneducated about the negative effects of alcohol. They lament a drunk wandering the streets. Then they are totally shocked when their annual routine blood test shows liver enzyme elevations from the three highballs they drank the night before their physical. They deplore the death toll from drunk drivers, but are careful to drive the back roads home after a dinner party. They are mystified when they develop burning in their feet during their late sixties and the neurologist makes a diagnosis of peripheral neuropathy, most often caused by chronic excessive alcohol intake.

I found it most interesting to learn that Philip Morris Corporation, a name made infamous in class action lawsuits for tobacco-related illness, owns Miller Brewing Company, producing some of the cleverest media campaigns ever for beer. The tobacco giant, fearing negative publicity from name recognition, asked its stockholders to approve a change to the Altria Group, an innocuous moniker for a mass killer who has simply changed weapons.

Motion pictures and television often glorify the world of intoxication rather than create an honest view of the risks of alcohol abuse. A trailer for a recent movie targeting the teen crowd chronicles a group of very cool snowboarders, and their excessive drinking is glorified. When one of the group passes out, they put him in his car, spin it around on the icy road, and then rouse him. He thinks he's really driving and panics while all his buddies fall down laughing. In another sequence, they all enormously enjoy watching a friend vomit because of excess drinking. With messages like these to our young people, how can we ever hope to bring home the real tragedy of alcoholism?

Stemming the tide of popular opinion and changing the perception of three generations of alcohol users is an enormous task. But small victories are being won. Faced with the knowledge that graduation night is the most dangerous night of a teen's life, parents and educators have joined forces to organize "sober grad night," all-night celebrations where kids are closely supervised and a variety of fun activities are substituted for the former oft-times drunken revels. New Year's Eve parties are being replaced by alcohol-free "First Night" celebrations in towns and cities nationwide. High schools have organized school-wide alcohol awareness campaigns where, in an assembly, the students view a mock-up of a drunk-driving collision. Emergency personnel minister to the victims, who are students of the school. One dies, and others are injured. The following day, the whole school attends the funeral and hears the parents and friends of the victim speak. Throughout the two days, an anonymous and silent representative of death appears in classrooms and removes students to represent the number of youth who are killed by alcohol each day.

It is an uphill battle. Creating an awareness of the physical, emotional, and spiritual damage that alcohol wreaks on our culture requires that we fight economic giants that reap huge revenues from the sale of alcohol. Wine grapes are the number-one agricultural revenue for my county of residence. Sales of alcoholic beverages reach into the billions of dollars. If the alcohol industry feels threatened by a changing public perception of their products, they will fight to maintain their markets.

Changes are possible, but we have to begin with the young. Once a pattern of alcohol abuse is established, it is very hard to alter. If we can keep kids from starting, we may be able to save lives. Perhaps a documentary revealing the tragic aspects of drinking could be required viewing for all high school students. If kids saw the devastation left in the wake of a drunk driver's path, watched an alcoholic die of ruptured esophageal varices, saw the mania of a violent drunk in lockup, heard the verbal abuse of a drunk spouse, or saw the bruises of a drunk-battered wife, maybe a few could say no. If we keep kids from starting, it would be a lot easier than getting them to quit. If someone had helped me question the normalcy of my parents' drinking as I was growing up, I might have seen my problem for what it was years ago. As I was, there are millions of young people at risk in this country today. It is worth a try to attempt to reach them. We owe them that.

BOB HAYES

September 30, 2002
To the Editor:

  Bob Hayes died last week. He was fifty-nine years old. He died of kidney failure due to complications from terminal cancer. He was an alcoholic and addicted to cocaine.

  Bob Hayes is the only man to own an Olympic gold medal and a Super Bowl ring. He was the fastest human for ten years. He won the Olympic gold medal in the 100-meter dash in the 1964 Tokyo Olympics and anchored the 4x100-meter relay team, taking the baton eight yards behind two other competitors and annihilating them at the finish.

  The Dallas Cowboys drafted him as a wide receiver, and he literally redefined the game. In those days, defensive backs could manhandle receivers, grabbing them and knocking them down, even past the five yards from scrimmage that is the rule today. But they couldn't catch Bob Hayes to knock him down. He was so fast that, after one fake, he was past the defensive back and in the clear, awaiting Roger Staubach's perfect spirals.

He had good hands, surprising for a man hired purely for his speed. And he had good moves once he caught the ball, eluding many frustrated safeties in the open field. In his first three seasons, he caught forty-six touchdown passes, a record that stood for two decades. He is still third on the all-time list.

If you ever saw him in a track singlet and shorts, you would think you had seen the perfect human body. With massive thighs and chiseled muscles, he was beautiful to look at.

But somewhere in the limelight of stardom, Bob Hayes found alcohol and cocaine. And they killed him. But before killing him, they ruined him. They reduced this most superb of human beings to a shell of his former self.

After fifteen years, losing battle after battle for sobriety, he finally got clean and sober, but the damage was done. I heard several interviews with him a few years before he died, which reflected his brain impairment from the drugs and alcohol. His speech was permanently slurred; the thought processes were infantile. It made me want to cry for this once-magnificent warrior. But that's what alcohol and drugs will do. They will destroy a body and a mind. Worst of all, they corrupt the spirit. They did it to Bob Hayes.

We mourn him. We shake our heads and say, "What a tragedy." But we, as individuals and society, do not acknowledge alcohol's potential for destruction. We glorify it. Coors has a new advertising theme, "Official Sponsor of Boys' Night Out." The images are of drunken revelry rife with implied sexual promiscuity. And that's cool. We are initiating a whole new generation of alcoholics. If they ever wake up to their addiction, they will have squandered two or three decades of their lives. If they are as unlucky as Bob Hayes, they may be permanently brain-impaired from drinking. They may lose their minds and their souls. When are we going to recognize the magnitude of this problem?

THE SOBERING TRUTH

10

ALCOHOL AND YOUR HEALTH: *THE GREAT HOAX*

It's not that you have been lied to. You've just been told a limited portion of the facts. The behemoth multinational corporations that market alcoholic beverages watch their stock prices soar every time a study is published demonstrating that alcohol is good for your health. And drinkers, many of whom are in denial that they have a problem or are in the early stage of alcoholism, can rationalize that their addiction is actually good for them. Is it really?

Mark Twain is quoted as saying that there are three kinds of falsehood: lies, damn lies, and statistics. So it is with data presented by the popular media regarding alcohol.

Narrowly defined, "moderate alcohol consumption" lowers health risk from cardiovascular disease. But it raises risk for various cancers, hepatitis, osteoporosis, immune suppression, accidents, and suicide. They don't tell you that part. With selective filtration of the facts, the liquor industry continues to advocate alcohol as a beneficial part of a healthful diet. Moderate and heavy drinkers, with denial and rationalization fully operational, proclaim alcohol to be the fountain of youth.

In stark contrast, the health hazards that tobacco use causes outrages the American public. Class action suits, public service announcements, prohibition of smoking in public places, and health warnings on packages attest to the increased public awareness and sentiment against tobacco use. Like alcohol lobbyists today, tobacco lobbyists at one time hid the devastating health risks from the public.

Alcohol is contributory to nine different types of cancer and gastroesophageal reflux disease (GERD). It is a leading cause of osteoporosis, suppresses the immune system, and is a major factor in highway deaths, spousal and child abuse, and homicide.

Smokers harm only themselves and their immediate family through secondhand exposure. Alcohol harms randomly on the streets and highways of America and, in an ever-widening circle, the family and friends of the alcoholic. So why doesn't the package labeling on alcoholic beverages really reflect the extent of these hazards? It does ... somewhat:

Government Warning: *(1) According to the surgeon general, women should not drink alcoholic beverages during pregnancy because of the risk of birth defects. (2) Consumption of alcoholic beverages impairs your ability to drive a car or operate machinery and may cause health problems.*

Why isn't the public better informed? Why isn't the warning more explicit? It's because of the power and money of the alcohol industry.

11

ALCOHOL AND CANCER

Let's start with a risk analysis of death at all stages of life. In youth, death rates are higher for accidents, suicide, homicide, and cancer than they are for heart disease. In middle age, the same is true, but cardiovascular disease is catching up. In old age, cardiovascular disease overtakes the other causes of death. Statistically, before the age of seventy-five, cancer and external causes of death are more common than heart disease. After seventy-five, heart disease becomes more important. Put simply, if we don't die of cancer, our heart is eventually going to give out.

With that background, let's examine the relationship between cancer and alcohol and carefully analyze the statistics and definitions used to perpetrate the great hoax that drinking alcohol is good for you.

The following were all patients of mine.

MOUTH CANCER

John was a strikingly handsome man when I first met him. Tall and lean, he was in his early sixties, and he had thick, black hair silvered at the temples, a warm smile, and a large hand with a firm but friendly handshake. But John had a perplexing problem, an unusual and difficult-to-treat form of oral cancer. Two years prior, his dentist had noticed an ominous-looking white patch on the inside of his left cheek. An oral surgeon had done a biopsy. The diagnosis was squamous cell carcinoma in situ.

The term "in situ" (literally translated "in place") is a concept that needs some explaining. When cancer begins in the skin (or the mucous membrane in the mouth), it begins in the top or cellular layer called the epidermis or mucosa, respectively. Here, cancer cells may first arise through mutation and then divide and grow into a colony of malignant cells. They are confined to the top layer, however, biologically fenced out by a tough little membrane beneath the epidermis/submucosa called the basement membrane. Before these cancer cells can invade into the deeper tissues, a new mutation has to occur in one of the cancer cells that produces an enzyme that can eat a hole in the basement membrane and allow the cells to invade. Without this enzyme, the cells are confined to the top layer and can grow for an indefinite period of time, "in situ." Thus, although imminently dangerous, such a proliferation of cells is precancerous.

So John had this patch on the inside of his cheek that showed in situ cancer. John's was squamous cell, a term that describes the flat platelike cells of the upper epidermis or mucosa. Because, most commonly, the cancer cells developing in any area of the body arise from normal cells that belong there, squamous cell cancer is the most common malignancy of the mouth. The word "carcinoma" is a Greek word that is synonymous with "cancer." They both mean "crab" and describe the gross appearance of a cancer as it spreads out into the tissues. The roots grossly resemble legs or claws invading into normal tissue from the main body of the cancer.

There are three main risk factors for squamous cell carcinoma of the mouth: tobacco, alcohol, and poor oral hygiene.

Surprisingly, John only had one factor, alcohol. He owned a very prestigious winery in our area, and he was a noted authority on wine. John never smoked, and his dental care was impeccable. So how did he develop oral cancer? It's because alcohol alone can cause it.

John had his carcinoma excised, but it wasn't three months after the sutures were removed that several new patches developed, one at the edge of the surgical scar and one on the inside of the other cheek. They both showed carcinoma in situ. Unfortunately, this is a common occurrence with oral cancer, as it is a multifocal disease. The negative influence that created the first cancer affected many other oral mucosal cells as well, and distinctly new lesions continue to arise.

Remarkably, John had no other risk factors than his wine drinking. And he was light-years away from being an alcoholic. But he tasted, sampled, and evaluated a lot of wine. At large tastings, he might sample two dozen wines. After evaluating the nose (fragrance), he would sip a small amount of a wine, swish it around, draw a small amount of air into his mouth, and experience the full flavor of the wine. By using this method of tasting, the wine spent a great deal more time in the mouth than if he were just drinking it.

John went to Stanford, where his cancers were excised and a large graft was placed on the inside of his cheek to cover the defect. As the graft healed, it contracted, shrinking his cheek down so he could barely open his mouth. On one of our follow-up visits, I could not insert a tongue depressor sideways between his teeth. I injected some steroid in the scar, and it loosened up enough to admit the tongue depressor, but just barely.

Radiation followed John's surgery, five days a week for seven weeks. His mouth grew so raw that he required a feeding tube to take nutrition. Two months after his final radiation treatment, two new patches were noted on the right cheek. Both were positive for cancer, and one was frankly invasive. Despite its removal, the cancer had spread to the lymph nodes beneath his jaw within six months. Radical neck surgery removed the nodes and some of the muscles of the right neck. Another course of radiation and chemotherapy produced a six-month remission, but a chest x-ray revealed several lung metastases, and severe hip pain led to a diagnosis of bony metastases in the pelvis. Within a year, John was dead. Drinking wine promoted the widespread metastatic disease that squamous cell carcinoma caused.

John's cancer was uncommon, but the wine had to have played a role. He had no other risk factors. As we will show later, bacteria in the mouth convert alcohol into cancer-causing acetaldehyde.

Although there are some back-page press reports and unobtrusive labeling of alcoholic beverages, the general public is not really aware that alcohol increases cancer risk. For a number of cancers, it does. Those cancers include the mouth, throat, esophagus, stomach, breast, liver, rectum, colon, prostate, and probably the pancreas. Interestingly, alcohol itself is not carcinogenic. You can bathe cells in tissue culture with alcohol, and it does not produce cancerous cells. You can feed alcohol to a bacterium called E. coli, as is done with other substances in a well-known cancer screening called the Ames test, and it will not produce mutations. But if you take the first metabolic breakdown product of alcohol, a substance called acetaldehyde, and incubate it with tissue culture cells or feed it to E. coli, it will produce cancer cells. So it appears that acetaldehyde is one of the culprits in alcohol's role as a cancer-causing drug.

It has been shown that bacteria in the mouth, stomach, and throughout the gastrointestinal tract are capable of producing acetaldehyde from alcohol. The acetaldehyde then bathes the epithelial cells, presumably creating mutations and producing the cancerous changes. Everyone who drinks alcohol presumably has increased amounts of acetaldehyde in their saliva, stomach secretions, and bowel. Why then, doesn't everyone develop cancer? A genetic predisposition apparently creates a wide variability among people in their ability to detoxify acetaldehyde. There is also a tremendous variability in how individual cells resist damage by acetaldehyde or repair the damage once it is done. The immune system also plays a key role in destroying cancer cells when they are at the one and two-cell stage.

The liver also produces acetaldehyde from alcohol that then circulates in the bloodstream throughout the body. So all the tissues are exposed to this carcinogen, but not at the high concentrations produced in the gut by bacteria. It's a wonder then that alcohol is not associated with increased cancer risks in all organs of the body. There are, however, some surprising facts about alcohol's role in tumor formation elsewhere in the body.

BREAST CANCER

Helen, a middle-aged housewife, had three grown children. She did not meet the definition of an alcoholic, but she and her husband regularly shared a glass or more of wine with dinner. She drank a bit more at weekend parties. Her gynecologist felt a breast lump on a routine exam despite the fact she had a normal mammogram ten months prior. A biopsy showed intraductal carcinoma. Excision of lymph nodes revealed that three of twelve nodes had microscopic spread of the tumor. She underwent radiation therapy and chemotherapy, and she has been on Tamoxifen for over three years now. To date, there is no evidence of recurrence of her breast cancer.

Helen had no family history of breast cancer. She had none of the other known risk factors for breast cancer, such as early onset of menstruation, having no children, having children later in life, failure to breast-feed, or hormone replacement therapy. She had three children in her twenties, breast-fed them all, and declined hormones after menopause. But she did drink alcohol regularly. Could that have played a role in developing breast cancer?

Surprisingly, the answer is yes. Several studies have shown an increase in breast cancer associated with alcohol intake. And these were not heavy drinkers. One study showed that women who drank one glass of wine a day had a 30 percent increase in breast cancer over a group that did not drink at all. The mechanism is not known, but perhaps breast tissue is more sensitive to the oncogenic ("onco" meaning "cancer" and "genic" meaning "to give rise to") effects of acetaldehyde.

In the recent past, reports that a specific hormone replacement therapy (Prempro) may slightly increase a woman's risk of breast cancer have caused a huge furor in the press. Millions of women have given up hormone replacement and face the risk of osteoporosis, atrophy (thinning) and increased sensitivity of vaginal tissue, and heart disease due to a seriously flawed study.[6] Concurrently, there is solid evidence that alcohol definitely increases the risk of breast cancer, yet you don't see these same women giving up their wine because they are unaware of alcohol's potential danger.

Breast cancer is on the increase, especially in First World countries. Could it be partially due to an increase in alcohol consumption in women? Yes, probably. In a startling recent study, it was found that women in upscale and affluent Marin County north of San Francisco have a 9 percent higher incidence of breast cancer than women in twenty-four other counties examined (Wrensch 2003,88-102). In addition, the rate of breast cancer was increasing 3.6 percent per year, six times higher than the national average. Looking at all the possible variables that may have contributed

---

[6] *This is according to my obstetrician-gynecologist friends.*

to the increase, researchers found that women who developed breast cancer were more likely to consume two or more drinks per day than were women in a control group who did not develop breast cancer.

So perhaps alcohol isn't so good for your health after all. But that's not what you hear from the wine marketers. They would have you think it is good for your health. If you are talking exclusively about cardiovascular health, it is. However, if you are talking about death from other causes, it is not.

COLON CANCER

Bill was in his mid-fifties, the picture of health. Lean and tan, he played on a basketball team at the local recreation league. He sold insurance, and he was quite successful. He was a moderate to heavy drinker, two glasses of wine with dinner on weeknights, a margarita and wine with dinner at weekend parties and during meals with clients. His only medical issue was a nagging problem with hemorrhoids since his late twenties. He had undergone two previous surgeries, so he just assumed it was another hemorrhoid when he developed new rectal bleeding. The bleeding wasn't too severe, and the memory of the painful removal was vivid. Bill would wait until the pain and bleeding were really disruptive before he would subject himself to another surgery.

When he had to wear diapers to keep from ruining his pants, he figured it was time. But he and his wife had booked a cruise to celebrate their twenty-fifth anniversary, so he postponed his doctor's appointment. He knew the proctologist personally from the country club, and he wasn't looking forward to the jokes in the locker room and the surgeon's rough technique. So his appointment was delayed another couple months.

Lying on the table, naked, and draped with a sheet, Bill felt embarrassed and incredibly vulnerable. He silently cursed his mother's side of the family, all of whom had hemorrhoids at a young age. Dr. Schultz's brusqueness left little room for tact or empathy. He groped around for a brief moment and then straightened up.

"This isn't any hemorrhoid. This is a tumor."

And it was. It was rectal cancer. Dr. Schultz did a biopsy and left a shocked patient to dress in silence and fear. The biopsy showed rectal cancer, a tumor the size of a pingpong ball. There was a flurry of tests. A CT scan showed a spread to the nodes of the pelvis.

Within a week, Bill had surgery. The tumor, rectum, and distal colon were removed. A colostomy was done, followed by two months of radiation and a year of chemotherapy. Despite aggressive measures, nodules of the tumor appeared in the liver and then in the lung. A different chemotherapy was tried to no avail. As Bill's liver filled with metastatic nodules, there was less healthy liver functioning to detoxify the ammonia and other toxins that the normal metabolism produced. Bill slowly slipped into a hepatic coma and died. He was fifty-six.

Did alcohol cause Bill's cancer? It contributed. Studies reveal there is an increase in rectal cancer in moderate to heavy drinkers. That is due in part to the acetaldehyde at work again on the cells of the rectal mucosa. There are other factors as well, including a high-fat diet.

PROSTATE CANCER

Jim was a single malt scotch drinker who loved his scotch. He had been having trouble with his urinary stream for several years. His PSA level[7] had been gradually climbing so his doctor referred him to a urologist. Six biopsies were done involving a not so pleasant process in which a probe is inserted into the prostate through the rectum. One of the biopsies showed an aggressive prostate cancer with a Gleason score of nine.[8] At forty-nine, Jim was young for prostate cancer, but, in some instances, younger men tend to have more aggressive tumors.

Jim had a radical prostatectomy. His PSA was zero for over a year, and then it began to creep up. A bone scan showed cancer in two vertebral bodies of Jim's spine. Radiation eliminated those metastases, but, six months later, a tumor was found in the humerus. Jim was started on a female hormone to suppress the tumor, causing his breasts to grow

---

[7] *PSA stands for prostatic sialic acid. Produced by prostate cells, it goes up in benign enlargement of the prostate and in cancer.*

[8] *The Gleason is determined by assessing the two most dominant cellular patterns in the biopsy, assigning them a number from one to five in order of increasing aggressiveness and adding them together. Gleason 9 prostate cancers are very aggressive.*

and his muscles to shrink. Subsequently, he had a seizure on the golf course. The resulting MRI revealed a tumor in his brain, But, before the neurosurgeon could operate, Jim began to turn yellow, and he was diagnosed with spread to his liver. He refused further treatment, slipped into a coma, and died. He was fifty-two.

Prostate cancer is epidemic in older men. It's the most common internal malignancy. Alcohol is at least partially responsible, specifically hard liquor. Beer and wine do not carry the same risk. In a study done of over seven thousand alumni of Harvard, a positive association was proven between moderate alcohol drinking and prostate cancer. Moderate consumers of hard liquor had a 61 to 67 percent increased risk of developing prostate cancer compared with men who consumed little or no alcohol. (Sesso 2001, 749-755)

Jim loved his scotch, but it seems like a high price to pay.

PANCREATIC CANCER

Carla felt as if she had the flu. She woke up in the morning nauseated and with a cramping pain in her belly. There was no fever, but she couldn't keep anything down. When her symptoms lasted a week, she finally went to the doctor. He ran some tests and called her the next day with a note of concern in his voice. He ordered a CT scan for the following morning. The scan showed a large, inoperable tumor in the pancreas. Carla got a second opinion at City of Hope, but they concurred. Chemotherapy was a possibility, but they were pessimistic about the chances for success. Miraculously, Carla's pancreatic cancer responded to chemotherapy. At this writing, she is well with a small but persistent tumor still present.

Pancreatic carcinoma is a leading cause of cancer-related deaths in this country. A direct link with alcohol consumption has not yet been established, although there is some strong incriminating evidence. Pancreatic cancers commonly have a peculiar gene rearrangement in a gene called K-ras. Such K-ras mutations have been correlated with alcohol consumption.

Not only does alcohol contribute to the development of cancers in many areas of the body, but, once a cancer has become established, no matter where it arose, there is evidence that alcohol may facilitate the spread of that cancer. The spread of a cancer from the primary site to new areas, both adjacent to and at distant sites from the primary, is known as metastasis ("meta" meaning "change" and "stasis" meaning "place"). Many factors affect the ability of a tumor to metastasize, but an important factor preventing such spread is a specialized immune cell, part of the T lymphocyte population called "natural killer T cells." These cells are like policemen patrolling your bloodstream and other tissues looking for trouble, searching for viruses, bacteria, fungi, yeast, and tumor cells. These cells are unique because they do not require previous immunization to a particular protein on the surface of a bacteria or tumor cell to work, and they are not specific for tumor or bacteria. They just attack anything that does not have the genetic profile of the host. These natural killer T cells (NKT cells) are extremely important in preventing metastasis. They patrol the body and attack and kill tumor cells spreading through the blood vessels and lymph system. Alcohol suppresses the number of functioning NKT cells in the body, promoting the spread of cancer to distant sites.

In a study using mice and experimental melanoma cells, mice with blood alcohol levels in the range of moderate to heavy alcohol use had a 50 percent depletion of NKT cells and an increase in metastases to the lung. As an aside, sunburn has also been shown to drastically reduce NKT cell numbers while vigorous exercise has been shown to increase NKTcell numbers.

So alcohol not only helps produce some cancers, but also promotes their spread. Not surprisingly, these facts are not publicized. The alcohol industry, a powerful lobby, would highly discourage the publication of this information. Unfortunately, the medical field has failed you as well. I know of no oncologists who advise their patients to abstain from alcohol once they have been diagnosed with cancer. I do.

My friend Scott developed squamous cell carcinoma, metastatic to his neck, twelve years after he quit smoking and drinking heavily. Despite aggressive surgery, radiation, and chemo, he lost a valiant battle. Having watched Scott suffer, I find it hard to read and listen to the propaganda about moderate alcohol being healthy.

In addition to the cancer-causing properties of acetaldehyde, the promotion of metastases due to the decrease in NKT cells and K-ras mutations, alcohol contributes to the development of cancers in another important way. There is a very important enzyme in many cells of the body, most importantly in the liver, called cytochrome p450. This enzyme is critical for the metabolism or processing of many substances in the body, especially breaking down drugs and detoxifying a variety of substances entering the body from the external environment. Alcohol induces a special variant of p450 called CYP 2E1, which, instead of detoxifying these chemicals, is responsible for changing some of them into carcinogens, thus producing a chemical environment conducive to the development of cancer. A number of substances known as pro-carcinogens are metabolized into carcinogens by CYP 2E1. Because alcohol increases the production of CYP 2E1, it results in higher concentrations of carcinogens as well.

In reviewing the medical literature on the health effects of alcohol, I found a Japanese study showing that drinkers died of all known forms of cancer more commonly than nondrinkers. Did you ever read that headline in your local newspaper? Did you hear it on the news? When a study demonstrating a health benefit of alcohol is published, it makes the front page. When a study proving that alcohol is a carcinogen is published, it is buried on the back pages, if it appears at all.

Twenty-five years ago, the health hazards of tobacco were just being defined, and the tobacco companies denied each new revelation. Now it is accepted fact that tobacco use is a serious health risk. The same is now becoming apparent of alcohol. There are serious cancer risks associated with its use. How long will it be before these facts are disseminated to the public and the marketers of this toxic substance own up to its cancer-causing potential?

If you are afraid of developing cancer and dying of it, you should not drink! If you have had cancer and you are afraid of a recurrence or metastasis, you should not drink!

12

HOW DOES ALCOHOL CAUSE CANCER?

In the past, there has been strong evidence that alcohol contributed to the causation of cancer. More recently, stronger evidence and an understanding of the actual mechanisms of causation have been determined. In addition, studies have shown that drinking alcohol may increase the likelihood of metastasis or recurrence of a previous cancer.

Let's look at the facts. Alcohol is known to cause cancer of the mouth, throat, colorectal area, esophagus, stomach, prostate, and breast. Canadian studies show that 3-6 drinks per week increases the recurrence of breast cancer. Canadian guidelines for safe alcohol consumption are one drink daily for women and two daily for men.

Alcohol is responsible for causing 100, 000 new cases of cancer every year in the US, and results in 20,000 deaths. Compare that to 13,500 deaths from alcohol-related traffic deaths. It is the third-leading cause of death in the US behind cigarette smoking and obesity.

Seventy percent of Americans drink alcohol. Only 45% of those are aware that drinking alcohol increases their cancer risk. Although the beneficial health effect of moderate drinking, especially wine, has been promoted, the risk of alcohol causing cancer outweighs the benefit of decreasing heart disease.

Smoking cigarettes and drinking alcohol increases the risk of cancer.

There are four ways alcohol causes cancer:

1) Alcohol does not itself cause cancer, but it is metabolized in the body to acetaldehyde which is a potent carcinogen. Acetaldehyde modifies cellular DNA, causing mutations and out of control cell division which produces cancers. Acetaldehyde partially does this by creating unstable chemicals called free radicals.
2) Alcohol alters hormone levels that increase cancer at hormone-sensitive sites like the breast and prostate.
3) Alcohol decreases levels of nutrients such as the B vitamins and folate that protect against cancer.
4) Alcohol acts like a solvent so that when it contacts other carcinogens it extracts and increases their concentration. This applies to cigarette smoking and particularly to smokeless tobacco.

Statistics back up the association of alcohol consumption with alcohol risk: At 80 years old, an individual who drank one or less alcoholic drinks per day has a 1% cancer risk.

Overall, women who drink one alcoholic drink or less per day have a 17% cancer risk, one drink per day a 19% risk, and two drinks per day a 22% risk.

Men: One or less drinks per day a 10% risk, one per day a 11% risk, and two drinks per day a 13% risk.

Women appear more vulnerable to the cancer-causing effect of alcohol. Their smaller size results in a more rapid rise in blood alcohol levels than men, increasing cancer risk.

Alcohol is known to alter hormone levels, accounting for the increase in breast cancer and prostate cancer in drinkers.

Smokers with cancer have an increased risk of metastatic disease if they drink alcohol.

Women with breast cancer have a higher risk of recurrence if they drink alcohol

Take it from the experts:

David Greenburg, M.D. Chief of Hematology and Oncology at Hackensack Meridian Jersey Shore Medical Center.

"If you play it by the book, you shouldn't drink any alcohol because it is toxic."

HOW DOES ALCOHOL CAUSE CANCER?

Why isn't there a warning label on alcoholic beverages about an increased risk of cancer?

Because it literally takes an act of Congress.

But, the Surgeon General of the United States, Vivek Murthy, MD issued an advisory on January 3, 2025 citing the increased cancer risk caused by alcohol and calling for an updated health warning on all alcoholic beverages.

THE SOBERING TRUTH

13

ALCOHOL AND THE HEART

George was blowing bubbles, but not Double Bubble or Bazooka and not the soapy stuff in the bottle. His bubbles were small and tinged with blood. George arrived at my medical admitting ward as a red blanket, a red sheet covering the gurney to denote his critical condition. He was desperately short of breath. His respiration was like the chug of a steam locomotive. Extremely agitated, he grabbed at my sleeve, pulling me toward him. He was experiencing one of the classical symptoms of advanced heart failure, the feeling of impending doom.

I went right to work. An oxygen mask was immediately fitted over his face, and rotating tourniquets were placed on his extremities to sequester some of the excess fluid to take the load off his heart. He was given morphine, furosemide (a powerful diuretic), and ouabain (a fast-acting digitalis), all intravenously. Within ten minutes, the medications were working. George was calmer. His respiratory and pulse rates were slowing. He had urinated over a liter. And he was no longer blowing bubbles. We saved him. But he would be back, as his heart was in terrible condition. He had alcoholic cardiomyopathy, a disease of the heart muscle caused by alcohol.

We are told that alcohol is good for the heart and it makes the heart healthier. But we are only told what they want us to know. It's a dosage thing. In small quantities, alcohol may be good for the heart, although, particularly with wine, it may not be the alcohol but another ingredient, resveratrol, that is beneficial. In higher dosages, alcohol is toxic to the myocardium (heart muscle). Over time, it may produce a severe weakening of the muscle that can result in a scenario that George and thousands of alcoholics like him experience up to five times before succumbing to congestive heart failure.

We are unaware of alcoholic cardiomyopathy because the alcohol lobby very carefully controls what appears in the national media about alcohol. What does appear often has a positive slant. Alcohol lowers your blood pressure, improves your memory, and decreases your cholesterol, and it is good for your heart.

The sound and print bites regarding alcohol in national media coverage are very carefully orchestrated. Papers from the prestigious *New England Journal of Medicine or Journal of the American Medical Association* are quoted, giving scientific credence to the claims of the benefits of drinking alcohol. All that appears is a two-line conclusion of a very complex study funded by a grant from some wine institute that may be flawed in its design. The headline states "Drinking Improves Heart Disease Survival." Excluded is that the study's definition of drinking is one glass of red wine (one and-a-half ounces of alcohol) a day, three times a week. HFAs who drank a liter of wine with dinner last night feel confident and smug that drinking is good for their health. But it isn't so. You need to hear the rest of the story.

The studies I note in this section on the health risks of alcohol are referenced at the end of the book by author. These citations represent just a small portion of the literature on the adverse health effects of drinking alcohol. None of them made headline news. None of them was funded by the liquor industry.

Let's get back to alcohol and heart disease. What are the facts? The landmark study cited as proof that alcohol promotes heart health is a study that compares the French with Americans. The study showed that France has a lower incidence of heart disease, although their diet is higher in fat, a contradiction christened "the French Paradox." A closer look revealed the French had a much higher consumption of wine than the Americans did. The initial conclusion was that consumption of alcohol, particularly in the form of red wine, was protective against the development of heart disease. Further study showed that a peculiar compound in the skin of grapes known as resveratrol might be the beneficial substance.

But there's more to the story that was never published. Let's call it the "French Conundrum." Although the French die less of heart disease, they succumb more frequently to cancer and suicide than Americans do. Why cancer? Researchers focused on this question and initially thought that resveratrol, which has mild estrogenic properties, was responsible. Further research has shown that resveratrol is anything but cancer-causing. On the contrary, the powerful antioxidant effect of resveratrol is preventive against cancer. So why is red wine associated with an increase in cancer? Acetaldehyde, the carcinogenic first breakdown product of alcohol, is more powerful than the cancer-preventing effect of the resveratrol. Recent studies show that as little as an ounce of alcohol daily is enough to increase cancer risk. With increasing amounts of alcohol, the increase is incremental. Anyone with scientific honesty can no longer dispute alcohol's carcinogenic effects. Why don't we hear more about it?

THE SOBERING TRUTH

14

ALCOHOL AND HYPERTENSION

Harold filled his third expensive prescription in three months. His blood pressure did not improve with the first two that had been prescribed, and now he was trying another.

Rightly so, he thought.

The first prescription rendered him temporarily impotent; the second one left him listless and bereft of any ambition. There's no telling how long he had high blood pressure. Harold was thirty-eight, and he hadn't seen a doctor for ten years before he recorded high readings at a blood donation drive. He was the first in his family to have hypertension, and it didn't make any sense. Or maybe it did.

Harold was a beer drinker. He drank three or four beers every night around dinner and maybe a six-pack or more on the weekends. He was not an alcoholic. He just liked his beer. After his diagnosis, he went online and researched the consequences of high blood pressure. They were more than a little frightening: kidney damage, eye damage, heart disease, stroke, ruptured aneurysm, and sudden death. That was enough to motivate him to control his hypertension. Hopefully, this new medication would work.

It might, but it would not eliminate the cause of the problem, and Harold might be destined to a lifetime of taking expensive medications with multiple side effects. It's ironic really when all he had to do was eliminate alcohol.

Even as little as one drink a day may increase blood pressure in men. Curiously, it takes increased consumption to cause the same problem in women. Millions of Americans spend billions of dollars yearly on hypertension medications, totally unaware that their wine with dinner or two beers watching the ball game was responsible for the problem. It is our goal to change that.

15

ALCOHOL AND DEPRESSION

Americans are depressed. Just look at the proliferation of antidepressants in the last several decades. Depression is a multimillion-dollar business in the United States and Europe. At least a third of the charts I open in my office have an antidepressant on the medication list.

The rapidly proliferating number of depressed individuals can be traced to planetary meltdown, economic uncertainty, widespread terrorism (both foreign and domestic), and a pandemic. The list goes on and on. Aging is depressing, as is illness. For a growing number of people, the world is a frightening place with random and chaotic tragedies. If they ever had faith in a providential wisdom, it is fading fast.

Besides pharmacologic help, many turn to alcohol. Somewhere in early experiences with drinking, people find there is a carefree euphoria that overcomes them during that first drink, caused by a decreased inhibition and anxiety in the earliest stages of intoxication. As our drinking progresses, subtle changes take place in the complex number and balance of the neurotransmitter chemicals in the brain, and we find we are uncomfortable without alcohol in our bloodstream, the beginning of dependence. The carefree moments are gone, but we keep trying, unaware the high is gradually being replaced by a low we don't understand and can't explain. After a while, we are no longer looking to feel good. Now we are trying to avoid feeling bad. We feel a psychic pain, much of which is produced by suppression of normal brain activity. The only thing that will relieve the pain is the thing that got us there in the first place. So we keep drinking. The progression gradually and subtly drops us into a deep, dark hole until we look around one day and there is no light, just this horrible feeling of depression and hopelessness.

How well I remember the few days before I hit bottom. I didn't really want that first beer, but I couldn't not drink it. After I did, I didn't feel any better, just pitiful and hopeless and beaten. I hated drinking, but I couldn't stop.

Alcohol is a depressant! You don't treat depression with a depressant!

16

ALCOHOL AND OSTEOPOROSIS

On the way to her garage, Gladys was walking down the back stairs with an armload of newspapers. She missed the second step and fell, landing hard. Her buttocks hit the concrete. She felt a blinding pain in her lower back, as if she had been slashed with a sword. She sat there for nearly an hour, paralyzed with pain, before her husband, Harold, came looking for her. He called 9-1-1, and Gladys was whisked to the emergency room of the local hospital. The attending physician immediately suspected the problem, as he had seen two similar cases in senior women that week. A back x-ray confirmed his diagnosis. Gladys had a compression fracture of her second lumbar vertebra. She had broken her back.

Gladys was suffering from osteoporosis ("osteo" means "bone" and "porosis" means "spongy"), an epidemic disease of seniors, particularly women. Insidious in its development, osteoporosis is caused by a loss or resorption of calcium from skeletal bone. As the result of the hard fall, the weight of her upper body literally collapsed a weakened second lumbar vertebra. An almost cube-like vertebral body that was originally two-and-a-half inches thick was now a little over an inch thick, causing severe pain (an eight or nine on the pain scale) that would last for several months.

Over the last fifteen years, I have watched my father become increasingly stooped over. Now, in his mid-eighties, he is so hunched in the upper back region that he is perpetually looking at the ground. It is not possible for him to straighten up, nor can he turn from side to side. He is literally a hunchback, with a male equivalent of the dowager's hump so commonly seen in women. The hump, caused by osteoporosis, results from demineralized bone shrinking and remodeling. The front of the vertebra is thinner than the back is, producing a forward bend. With time, the disc spaces between the vertebrae can be obliterated, and the vertebrae actually fuse.

As I watched this occur in my father, I was surprised by its severity and progression and mystified as to its cause. My dad had been a heavy smoker, one recognized cause of osteoporosis, but I knew many male smokers who didn't have the degree of osteoporosis seen in my dad. Although medium in height, he was a large-boned, muscular man, the last person in whom you would expect osteoporosis.

Then, as I researched the health effects of alcohol, I came across a reference in the literature that astonished me. Alcohol is a leading cause of osteoporosis. My dad's heavy drinking and smoking created an osteoporosis double whammy.

The baby boomer generation, now approaching late middle age, is a fertile ground for the development of osteoporosis. Forty percent of women in their fifties have osteopenia, a decreased level of calcium in the bone that is an intermediate step to osteoporosis. The estimates are that fully half of adult women in America develop osteoporosis in their lifetime. The critical skeletal areas affected by osteoporosis are the vertebrae and hip. The head of the femur, a large ball-like bone that fits into the hip socket, is connected to the vertical shaft of the femur by a relatively narrow bone called the neck, which attaches at almost a right angle. Here, the hip typically fractures through an osteoporotic neck of the femur.

It certainly came as a surprise to me, a doctor, that alcohol was a leading cause of osteoporosis. It is not common knowledge in the general population, let alone in the medical community. With all the information about diet, exercise, and hormone replacement in the press and self-help magazines, one would think somewhere there might be a mention of alcohol's contribution to this ubiquitous disease of the elderly.

Alcohol causes osteoporosis by lowering the amount of calcium in the bloodstream via two mechanisms:

- Alcohol is a diuretic, increasing urine production by the kidney. Calcium and magnesium are passively carried out with the increased urine flow.
- Ingestion of alcohol decreases the production of parathyroid hormone. This hormone, produced by several pea-sized glands located adjacent to ("para") the thyroid gland, causes calcium levels to rise in the blood by increasing absorption from the gut and decreasing kidney excretion of calcium. When alcohol is ingested, the calcium level in the blood drops, and the urinary excretion of calcium increases. These changes are maximized eight to twelve hours after intake. Thus, people who drink on a daily basis are chronically depriving their bones of calcium.

Does alcohol consumption in the elderly account in part for the increase in osteoporosis and its morbidity? Absolutely!

THE SOBERING TRUTH

## 17

ALCOHOL AND THE IMMUNE SYSTEM

Helen was a former army nurse. She drank bourbon straight up every night, and she didn't care who knew it. She was as tough as an old shoe, ran her ward at LA County like her army hospital, and didn't take any guff from anybody, especially any smartass intern. I liked her immediately. With Helen, there were no pretenses. And she liked me because I treated her with the deference she deserved after thirty years of nursing. Conversely, she made life miserable for one member of my internship team, an arrogant young doctor named Rob Heller. The son of a doctor, a silver spooner, Rob belittled the nurses and always insisted on being called "Doctor Heller."

Helen had seen his type and problem before. He had a severe case of chronic self-importantism. And she had the cure. She would wait until he had just settled into his bunk in the sleeping room to call him for a problem patient who hadn't had a bowel movement in three days. Then Doctor Heller would have to get up, put on a glove, and de-impact the poor old lady, removing concrete-like nodules of stool from her rectum. By contrast, Helen would always let me know when the IV on one of my patients was causing problems so I could retape it or flush it out before it was useless. With Doctor Heller, she waited until the IV had infiltrated or was hopelessly plugged. Then she told him, necessitating its replacement. Helen was a piece of work! In a month on her service, I'll bet Rob didn't get more than twenty minutes of sleep the nights that we were on call.

But Helen always seemed to be sick. Coughing, wheezing, and blowing her nose every five minutes, she carried one of those small packages of Kleenex in her coat pocket and replenished it two or three times a night from a large carton in her desk drawer. Helen caught every cold that came onto the wards. Because she had been exposed to illness and disease her entire career, one would think she'd be immune to every virus on earth, but the opposite was true.

Only years later did it make sense to me. It was the whiskey. Alcohol suppresses the immune system. Upper respiratory viruses are foreign invaders. When they reach the nasal passages or throat, a small army of immune defenders is supposed to meet them. The virus may be confronted by a Langerhans cell, a modified histiocyte, which interacts with the virus, recognizing foreign proteins on its surface and presenting them to T lymphocytes. T lymphocytes, once activated, give off complex and sophisticated chemical messages that recruit other immune cells. Eventually, in about ten to fourteen days, they produce antibodies that neutralize the invading virus. This takes time. Meanwhile, the virus is replicating and causing the host to be sick.

Another platoon of the immune army doesn't need time to fight back. Natural Killer T (NKT) cells nonspecifically attack any non-host proteins, whether they be on viruses, bacteria, fungi, or tumor cells. They may completely inactivate invading viral particles and prevent an infection even before the more robust but delayed immune system gets into the act.

There is a catch. Several physical stimuli influence the number and vigor of NKT cells. Vigorous exercise has been shown, for instance, to increase the number of NKT cells, yet alcohol decreases them significantly. That means that viruses attacking the host have time to multiply before the delayed system can muster the troops. The patient becomes ill.

So it's no wonder Helen was always sick. The liquor did it to her. By decreasing the number of NKT cells, Helen was made more vulnerable to every virus that was coughed across her desk. And even more importantly, those same NKT cells are one of our most important defenders against cancer, probably destroying mutant cells before they have a chance to develop into significant tumors. So, not only was Helen sick all the time, but she bore a higher risk of developing cancer as well.

18

ALCOHOL AND ALLERGIES

Ron lives with two inhalers as constant companions. He has had asthma since he was a young child. At times, it has been severe and unrelenting. Despite that, Ron excelled as a high school and college cross-country runner and horseman. He is also a fine golfer. In recent years, however, the asthma has worsened, making him even more dependent on his inhalers and several pills that he takes to lessen the symptoms. He has experienced a lot of work stress as he climbs his way up the corporate ladder, and I always attributed his worsening to that. Imagine my surprise when, in the course of my research on the health effects of alcohol, I discovered that alcohol greatly aggravates allergies of all kinds, including asthma.

Allergies are a major cause of discomfort and disability for over a third of the population. They manifest as asthma, hay fever, eczema, and food allergies. Recent studies indicate that allergies are on the rise in the United States.

An abnormal antibody, present only in people with allergies, causes these diseases. The antibody is called immunoglobulin E (IgE). IgE does not occur in normal, nonallergic people unless they are infested with parasites, such as intestinal worms. There is some evidence that IgE may help defend against and destroy such parasites, but, when they are gone, the IgE levels drop to a negligible level. In allergic people, however, the IgE levels are almost always high. They are specifically developed against certain substances, known as allergens, like grass pollen in the case of hay fever or peanuts in the case of food allergies. Allergists actually test patients for specific allergies by assaying the level of IgE in their blood that reacts to these substances.

The immune system, even when it malfunctions, is a marvel. Each individual IgE molecule is specific for a unique allergen. The IgE molecule for peanuts will not respond to the protein allergen in almonds, pecans, or any other nuts. The specific molecule of IgE has a receptor on its surface that is composed of a series of amino acids that is unique to that allergen. The receptor, extending out from the surface of the IgE molecule, is like a trailer hitch. It will only fit a similar hitch on the trailer. The receptor has to be just the right size and shape to attach to the allergen. When the correct allergen is present, the receptor and allergen fit together like a lock and key or cup and ball of the trailer hitch. Once the receptor docks with the allergen, the fused proteins react with a feisty little cell known as a mast cell, which is present throughout the body, to produce allergy symptoms. The aroused mast cell releases small granules stored within it that contain proteins that produce intense inflammation. Notable among these are histamine, bradykinin, and a pesky little protein called slow-reacting substance of anaphylaxis. Histamine causes intense itching, redness, and swelling of the skin and a spasm of the tiny muscles that encircle the airways in the lungs, causing the narrowing or constriction of the bronchioles so characteristic of asthma.

Most of our treatments for these allergic problems target the histamine and other mediators of inflammation. We treat itching with antihistamines and swelling and inflammation of eczema and asthma with cortisone-like steroids that diminish the inflammation. But we are treating the results of the abnormal reaction after it happens, slamming the barn door after the horse is long gone. Our therapeutic efforts need to be focused on decreasing IgE production or blocking its reaction with the allergen. The latter is currently being developed. In Europe, proteins called blocking antibodies are being used that attach to IgE molecules and prevent them from seeking out their allergen. Chronic hives are being treated with some success by this strategy, and the future looks bright for this kind of treatment.

Reducing IgE is also an excellent rationale for diminishing allergic illness. Because one of the potent stimulants to IgE production is alcohol, abstaining from drinking should greatly reduce allergic symptoms in susceptible individuals. Speaking from personal experience, it does. I have one-tenth the sneezing and itchy, watery eyes in the spring than I had before I quit drinking. Part of that is attributable to eliminating alcohol. The rest is due to my intake of large doses of vitamin E, which has also been shown to decrease IgE production. Additionally, IgE has a life span of ninety days in the bloodstream, so it requires a long-term commitment to realize a reduction of allergic symptoms.

Have you ever heard that alcohol increases allergy problems? Probably not. The conspiracy of silence by alcohol producers publicizes only the health benefits of alcohol, not the legion of illnesses and malignancies promoted by its use.

THE SOBERING TRUTH

19

ALCOHOL AND GERD

Wayne thought he was dying. Sweat poured off his forehead as pain gripped him, deep in the middle of his chest. He couldn't lie down. This was the third time this week, and the nitroglycerin failed to help. He couldn't get his breath. Certain he was having a heart attack, he called 9-1-1. The paramedics were there within five minutes. Everything was a blur. Almost instantly, they had put an oxygen mask over his face, taken his blood pressure and pulse, hooked him up to an electrocardiogram telemetry system, started an IV, and placed him on a gurney and into their unit. He was a Code 3 to Mar Vista Hospital. There, after three hours of cardiac monitoring, blood tests to assess heart muscle damage, morphine, and oxygen, the emergency room staff concluded it was not a heart attack. Rather, it was pain coming from the upper esophagus, badly irritated by acid contents that leaked back from a faulty valve at the opening to the stomach. Previously called heartburn, a fairly accurate description, the condition is now referred to as gastroesophageal reflux disease (GERD). It is common and on the increase.

Wayne has GERD. The corrosive contents of his stomach, rife with enzymes powerful enough to auto-digest his own tissues and hydrochloric acid strong enough to dissolve the toughest gristle on a porterhouse steak, leak back into the esophagus and burn it. The mucosa (lining) of the esophagus wasn't designed to withstand that chemical insult. The burn results in erosion of the mucosa, exposing the delicate collagen of the submucosa and smooth muscle beneath it. Just like an acid burn on the skin, it heals with scarring. With repeated episodes, the scarring infiltrates and replaces the muscle. The complex and precise process of peristalsis (bands of smooth muscle encircling the esophagus gently milk food downward from mouth to stomach) is permanently impaired. The lower end of the esophagus becomes atonic (unmoving). The essential muscular valve separating the esophagus from the stomach (cardioesophageal sphincter) is destroyed. The process gradually worsens, resulting in a scarred and rigid esophagus that doesn't function at all.

The enormous popularity of drugs that decrease stomach acid production is testimony to the widespread occurrence of GERD. These drugs are advertised heavily on television, an interesting twist on the marketing strategy of pharmaceutical companies:

- Don't advertise to the doctors.
- Advertise to the patients.
- Then they will solicit the drug from their physicians.

Wayne has to wait at least two hours after eating before he can lie supine, enough time to allow the stomach to fully empty so there are no corrosive contents to backflow into the esophagus. He is not alone. Millions of Americans with GERD rationalize it is the stress of the modern world, and the bizarre eating schedules that demanding work schedules necessitate that increase the acid production in their stomachs. Doctors' orders to restrict their drinking go unheeded. They continue to consume the highball after work and the two or three glasses of wine with dinner followed by Prevacid or Tagamet. They eat and drink it all and then pop the fix-it pill.

In large part, alcohol causes GERD. Alcohol causes a relaxation of the cardioesophageal sphincter, which allows the acid contents of the stomach to reflux into the lower esophagus and burn it. Alcohol also impairs the motility or muscle action of esophageal peristalsis. The combination of drinking alcohol and lying down with a stomach full of food, acid, and digestive enzymes is the formula for creating GERD.

Wayne is happy now. He takes his Prevacid regularly so he can eat and drink anything he wants without trips to the emergency room. Pharmaceutical companies are profiting, and we continue, for the most part, to be unaware of alcohol's role in the GERD epidemic.

20

ALCOHOL AND PERIPHERAL NEUROPATHY

Florence's muscular body and quick mind belie her eighty-two years of age. She plays golf twice a week and volunteers at the hospital. But she complains bitterly of a burning sensation in her feet that is steadily worsening, comparable to walking on a bed of hot coals.

Florence suffers from peripheral neuropathy. The sensory nerves to the skin of her feet are damaged. Like wires with frayed insulation, the electrical messages carried in these nerves frequently short-circuit, causing the nerves to report abnormal sensations or feelings that aren't really there. The result is a combination of numbness, tingling, or burning that occurs in the lower legs and feet, especially on the soles. Present all the time, it is most distressing at night when many other sensory stimuli diminish. What had been slightly annoying warmth on the bottoms of the feet during the day becomes an intolerable, searing pain at night. Unfortunately, this is an increasingly common problem for our senior population.

Three major causes of peripheral neuropathy are diabetes, nutritional deficiencies, and alcohol consumption. Oftentimes, there is no identifiable cause, and it is written off as aging nerves. Alcohol probably causes many of these cases, but the investigating doctor is not getting an adequate idea of how much the patient drinks or used to drink, as many alcoholic patients lie about their habit.

Alcohol causes nerve damage by at least two mechanisms:
- It is a cell poison, damaging and killing nerve cells in the brain and spinal cord. With the death of peripheral nerve cells or neurons, there is a decreased sensation in the involved areas. If the nerves are damaged, they function abnormally and may report back peculiar sensations such as itching, tingling, or burning.
- Alcohol also produces nerve damage as it may cause a deficiency of several vitamins that are essential for neuronal function. People who drink heavily often do not pay attention to eating well. Alcoholic calories take the place of good nutrition. When a person is intoxicated on a regular basis, he may not include the major food groups in every meal. For some heavy drinkers, the three major food groups may be beer, wine, and whiskey. As a result, foods with critical vitamins for healthy nerve function may be omitted.

Folic acid, thiamine (B1), and vitamin B12 are thought to be critical for healthy nerve function. Not surprisingly, many alcoholics show low levels of these vitamins in their bodies, and their neuropathies are indistinguishable from those produced by these deficiencies.

With an aging population, peripheral neuropathy is becoming more of a health problem. Many cases due to neuronal degeneration related simply to the aging process may not be preventable with our current medical knowledge. But many cases related to the chronic abuse of alcohol are. We need to get the word out.

21

ALCOHOL AND INSOMNIA

Brenda hasn't had a good night's sleep in twenty years. She attributes it to the stress of her work as a legal secretary for a very demanding boss and raising two boys as a single parent. Sleep deprivation adds to the stress, shortening her fuse with her kids and coworkers.

Brenda falls asleep promptly when retiring and sleeps soundly for four hours. Then she awakens, tossing and turning while thinking about the bills, her ex-husband's delinquency with the child support, and the contracts she prepared for her boss that day. She doesn't sleep the rest of the night. She would never suspect that it might be the two glasses of wine she has before and during dinner to relax.

Alcohol depresses nerve function, both in the brain and throughout the nervous system. This alcohol, although a relatively small amount, is enough to alter the delicate chemical balance in the brain. With the depression of nerve function, the alcohol produces a mild sedative effect, and the initiation of sleep comes easily. But when the three to five ounces of alcohol are completely metabolized,[9] there is a rebound hyperactivity of the nerves. This produces wakefulness and persists long enough to ruin a good night's sleep.

Alcohol also reduces rapid eye movement (REM) sleep, a stage of sleep associated with dreaming, thought to be important for resting and recharging one's emotional energy. Many regular drinkers consequently

---

[9] *The liver can metabolize one to one-and-a-half ounces per hour.*

experience a diminution in the amount and quality of restfulness of their sleep.

Recovering alcoholics may experience months of insomnia as the brain overreacts to the absence of the depressant effect of alcohol. My friend Bud had a year of sleeplessness following his recovery.

In the most severe form, this reflex hyperactivity of the brain following withdrawal of alcohol produces a severe reaction, delirium tremens, commonly called DTs. Within hours of removal of alcohol, the abstinent alcoholic begins to tremble and then shake. This is the rebound hyperactivity of motor nerves, so long depressed by alcohol. In the most severe cases, the muscular hyperactivity will progress to grand mal seizures, or rum fits. Untreated, they may be fatal.

The sensory nerves, no longer depressed, report all manner of unusual sensations, including itching, burning, or aggravating feelings like ants crawling on the skin. The higher centers of the brain go haywire. Abstinent alcoholics are confused, having no grasp on reality and no orientation in time and space. Visual and auditory hallucinations are common.

Alcoholics who have suffered serious withdrawal untreated never want to repeat the experience. The least bit of shaking necessitates a stiff drink to get the blood alcohol level up quickly and bathe those neurons with the two-carbon depressant to which they are habituated. It is a depressingly realistic way of life for many chronic alcoholics.

22

ALCOHOLIC ENCEPHALOPATHY

Reuben was back again. I could see the polished mahogany top of his bald pate on the gurney and bright yellow of the fluid in his IV. They spiked his D5W (5 percent dextrose in water) with Berocca-C, a mix of B vitamins with vitamin C. It was a taxicab yellow fluid clearly indicating to any passing medical staff that the patient was a severe chronic alcoholic. Reuben had such severe deficiencies that he had almost died twice.

Reuben suffered from Wernicke's encephalopathy, an intense disruption of brain function due to vitamin deficiencies caused by severe alcoholism. The B vitamins, in particular thiamine (B1), are critical enzymes in the metabolism of glucose. Unlike other parts of the body, which can metabolize fats and proteins, the brain and spinal cord can only burn glucose for fuel. That's why low blood sugar causes loss of consciousness and grand mal seizures. Alcoholics are deficient in B vitamins for three reasons:

- They ingest many of their calories from alcohol, neglecting their intake of vitamins.
- They require more B vitamins than nonalcoholics because their daily intake of alcohol requires additional B vitamins to metabolize.
- Chronic alcoholism reduces the production and absorption of many vitamins from the intestine, including the B vitamins.

Wernicke's encephalopathy has a 20 percent fatality rate in emergency rooms. Brain and spinal cord cells (neurons) are very unhappy when they don't have enough glucose. In mild to moderate deficiency states, they malfunction, but the damage is reversible. In severe chronic cases, the neurons die, resulting in permanent injuries.

Reuben was a textbook example of the manifestations of severe chronic thiamine deficiency as they affect the central nervous system. Neuronal injury in the cerebrum or higher centers of the brain produced confusion, disorientation, and a severe loss of memory. I had admitted Reuben twice before, and he had no recollection of me or what day or month it was. He also had been admitted twice in coma, but the Berocca-C had revived him both times.

Involvement of Reuben's cerebellum, the balance and coordination centers of the brain, produced a staggering broad-based gait (when he could walk) and inability to do simple things such as touching his nose with his fingertip (How could he get a bottle to his mouth?). Reuben's cranial nerves were severely involved, as is often the case. Damage to the muscles that control facial expression, eye movement, and vision caused partial paralysis of his eye muscles, particularly the abductors (those that look to the sides), so his eyes were continually crossed. Imbalance and weakness of his eye muscles also created a twitching movement of the eyeball called nystagmus. Temporary horizontal nystagmus is a sign of acute intoxication that police officers use when they do field sobriety tests. Reuben's nystagmus was horizontal and vertical, and it was permanent.

Reuben also had involvement of peripheral nerves causing a polyneuropathy involving numbness, tingling, and burning. Interestingly, peripheral neuropathy, relatively common in seniors, is indistinguishable from alcohol-induced neuropathy. It is possible that many such cases result from heavy social drinking.

Reuben recovered again with Berocca-C. But he died a month later on a similar admission of heart failure. The sympathetic nerves, which control the tiny muscles in the body's blood vessels, were damaged beyond repair. This caused the muscles to relax, creating a massive dilation of blood vessels. The heart can't pump fast enough to fill such a vastly increased vascular volume. Shock and death ensued.

The shiny brown pate and lifesaving bottle of Berocca-C were gone.

But the lessons he taught a whole decade of medical students and interns about alcohol deficiency states and the catastrophic effect on the brain were not lost on this student.

A description and discussion of the most devastating effects of alcohol on the brain and spinal cord might seem out of place in this book. But if alcohol is toxic to neurons and a lot of alcohol does a huge amount of damage, isn't it logical that low-level injury on a long-term basis would produce significant damage as well? Is the peripheral neuropathy seen increasingly in seniors due to heavy social drinking? Is the unsteadiness of old age in part due to cerebellar damage from alcohol? Is the cognitive impairment and memory loss so prevalent in seniors due, in part, to chronic alcohol toxicity?

The answers are probably yes. In a recent study of the elderly, more brain atrophy (shrinkage), as manifested by enlargement of fluid-filled spaces in the brain called ventricles, was seen in drinkers than in nondrinkers (Enzinger 2005). This is incriminating evidence, relegated to the back pages of the daily news.

THE SOBERING TRUTH

23

ALCOHOLIC HEPATITIS

Bart was quite upset when the blood bank refused to allow him to donate blood because of what they called his hepatitis. A man in his mid-fifties, Bart has been a regular blood donor since his late twenties. His name appears on the five-gallon donor plaque, and he aspired to have it on the ten-gallon plaque as well. There's no chance now as the blood bank will no longer accept him as a donor. His liver enzymes were elevated in last month's blood sample. Bart has since been to his personal physician, and he had a comprehensive panel of blood tests. He was negative for hepatitis A, B, and C; mononucleosis; and HIV, but the blood bank still refuses his blood. They can't risk giving a patient a unit of blood that may contain an infectious form of hepatitis as yet unknown. Having transmitted hundreds of thousands of cases of hepatitis C and HIV to unwitting blood recipients before adequate screening tests were developed, blood banks are now very cautious. There are other strains of HIV and hepatitis for which we have no adequate tests to date, so it's safer to exclude those individuals who have elevated liver enzymes from the donor pool. Bart will never make the ten-gallon club, but not because he has a new strain of hepatitis. His drinking has increased lately, resulting in elevated liver enzymes on the screening test for his last unit of donated blood.

Alcohol is a cell poison, as is acetaldehyde, the first breakdown product in the metabolism of alcohol. Even in small doses, alcohol injures and kills liver cells, causing them to leak the enzymes that enable them to process digested material such as proteins, fats, and carbohydrates and detoxify harmful substances that have been ingested. Liver enzymes can be measured in a blood sample. When they are elevated from the normally low levels, it means the liver is suffering some ongoing damage. The general term for any inflammation of the liver is hepatitis. The term does not imply an infectious origin, although people interpret it that way. It actually denotes any process that results in injury to liver cells with the attendant inflammation. The various forms of hepatitis that are caused by microorganisms are labeled infectious hepatitis.

Every time Bart has a glass of wine, he has a small episode of hepatitis. Liver cells are injured, and some die, releasing their enzymes. The liver is a remarkably resilient organ. As much as 90 percent of the liver can be surgically removed. The remainder will, in part, regenerate. But with alcohol and other substances that are toxic to the liver, it is not analogous to removing a hunk of liver and leaving a healthy piece to regenerate. Rather, alcohol causes diffuse injury and death to liver cells, resulting in the formation of fibrosis (scar tissue). Fibrosis changes the very complex and intricate way in which the liver functions. The liver cells, bile ducts, and portal veins are all arranged in a precise manner so the liver can do its job of metabolizing nutrients and detoxifying harmful substances both formed within the body (ammonia) and introduced extrinsically (drugs, environmental toxins, or alcohol). The fibrosis that results from alcohol injury to liver cells alters this intricate architecture so different component cells don't hook up properly to do their job. The short-term result is a liver that is compromised in its ability to perform its jobs. The long-term result is a liver that develops the extreme form of fibrosis known as cirrhosis, rendering it incapable of functioning efficiently and resulting in liver failure with its myriad medical complications.

Drinking is such a socially acceptable and culturally ingrained activity that most people ignore its contribution to serious liver damage. Patients who are wary of taking certain medications because they have a risk of causing liver damage always amuse me. A very effective oral medication for athlete's foot and toenail fungus, for instance, has a chance of producing liver toxicity in one-tenth of 1 percent of the people who take it. The hepatitis is mild to moderate and completely reversible when the drug is stopped. And yet, when I present to patients the option of taking this drug, at least half will say, "Oh no, doctor. I don't want to take anything that has a risk of damaging my liver." Many of these same patients had two highballs before dinner and split a bottle of wine with their spouse the night before, unaware that the damage caused by alcohol has the same potential seriousness as that caused by medication. Some more addicted patients are unwilling or unable to restrict their alcohol intake while taking antifungal medication.

Do other medications cause hepatitis? Yes. Medications with potential liver toxicity include those prescribed for high blood pressure, high cholesterol, seizure disorders, cardiac arrhythmias, and arthritis. Blood thinners, antibiotics, and other prescription drugs can also affect liver function. Conscientious physicians usually discuss potential side effects with their patients before they prescribe medications. The patient listens attentively and reassures the doctor that she only has a glass of wine with dinner and will abstain. She does for a while. But when she has a couple glasses of champagne at a wedding with no reaction, she adds a glass of wine with dinner. Five years after the medication was prescribed, she has forgotten the admonition about drinking. She is ingesting two hepatotoxic (liver-toxic) substances. If she is taking additional medication, she may be ingesting even more.

Alcoholism is epidemic in our senior population. A significant number of seniors are bored or depressed. Oftentimes, they have suffered a loss, and they are grieving. Many are in chronic pain from arthritis or back problems. As a result, seniors tend to drink or drink more, although alcohol enhances depression instead of improving it. And it is a lousy pain medication.

In due time, seniors no longer drink for pain relief, depression, or a pick-me-up. Now they drink because they cannot stop. Unwittingly, they have learned the truth about alcohol. It is powerfully addictive.

THE SOBERING TRUTH

24

ALCOHOLIC PANCREATITIS

It started with dry heaves. Dan had been hitting it pretty hard over the weekend, and he just thought it was part of the hangover package. When the pain and fever began, he decided he must have had the flu. Then all hell broke loose. The pain was like nothing he had ever experienced or imagined. It was boring through him, like someone pushing a white-hot branding iron through his belly. He kept vomiting. Initially, it was nothing. Then it was a bitter yellow that he thought must be bile. Then it was yellow with flecks of blood.

He was frantic with pain. He called 9-1-1. The paramedics didn't waste any time. They had vital signs, an IV started, and EKG leads on him within several minutes. They had him at Mercy Hospital within ten. There the waiting began, followed by the probing, testing, and ultrasound. They gave him some morphine to take the edge off the pain, but it was still unbearable. Four hours after the first heave, the emergency room doctor gave Dan the news. He was having an attack of pancreatitis brought on by the weekend bender.

The pancreas, a fair-sized organ, lies horizontally across the back of your abdominal cavity, just below the diaphragm.

It is such a tireless and usually trouble-free organ that its purpose is hardly known to the layperson. The majority of the gland is made up of aggregates of cells that make and secrete enzymes that are responsible for digesting the food we eat. A much smaller portion is made up of islands of cells that make important hormones for controlling our blood sugar, insulin and glucagon. The digestive enzyme portion is the major player in pancreatitis. For reasons that are still not known, alcohol causes severe inflammation in the pancreas. Cells containing precursors of digestive enzymes fall apart, the precursors are converted to the active enzymes, and the pancreas digests itself instead of digesting the food in the intestine. What follows is a chain reaction:

- More enzymes are released, killing more gland and so on until it burns itself out or
- The entire gland becomes involved, resulting in massive inflammation, shock, and death.

In the United States, alcohol causes fifty percent of pancreatitis attacks, but the exact mechanism remains a mystery. The results of the attacks are no mystery. Death of the pancreatic cells causes massive inflammation. If the patient survives, the pancreas may scar, reducing its ability to digest food and producing malabsorption. Sufficient scarring can also reduce the amount of insulin the pancreas secretes, resulting in diabetes. Large holes can be digested in the pancreas, leaving pseudocysts that can ferment infection and impair function. Frequently, even if the patient abstains from alcohol, the attacks continue for a lifetime. Despite the relative obscurity of pancreatitis in the public consciousness, it was found in 0.5 percent of all autopsies in a large American regional hospital. Many who survive the attack wish they had been one of those statistics.

Dan survived his horrendous attack of pancreatitis. Two weeks of hell included a tube down his nose draining his stomach, IV feeding, and pain beyond his comprehension, only partially relieved by the most potent narcotics. His insulin-producing cells were one of the casualties of his overindulgence. He is now an insulin-dependent diabetic, giving himself three injections per day. He left the hospital totally changed, shocked by the physical alterations the attack had brought on and frightened it could happen again at any time. And it could.

Pancreatic cancer has been in the news lately as a few high-profile people have succumbed to it. Although not directly linked, there is some strong indirect evidence that alcohol plays a role in pancreatic cancer's development.

25

ALCOHOL, OBESITY, AND DIABETES

The love handles and beer belly were impressive. Harry was in for a long-overdue checkup, and his mid-fifties frame was woefully overburdened. At five-foot-eleven and two hundred and twenty pounds, Harry had a list of medical problems that read like a litany of risk factors for an early demise, including hypertension, coronary artery disease, diabetes, and elevated triglycerides. In actuality, he had only one problem. He drank too much.

The body treats alcohol as if it were a sugar, or a simple carbohydrate. A can of beer, often referred to as a "liquid sandwich," tallies one hundred and fifty calories of pure carbohydrates. When you drink a six-pack of beer, it's similar to eating nine hundred calories of sugar, but instead of a sugar high, you get intoxicated.

Carbohydrates are the high-octane fuel of the body. The muscles use them for strenuous exercise. Glucose, the simplest of the carbohydrates, is the sole usable source of energy for the brain. The body has a limited ability to store carbohydrates. It packs away a little in muscles for a burst of energy in emergencies, and it stores some in the liver. In both venues, carbohydrate is stored in a long chain of glucose molecules linked together called glycogen. Any excess carbohydrate the body is unable to burn for its daily energy requirement is converted into fat. Long chains of carbohydrates are converted into fat and attached to a three-carbon molecule called glycerin, producing triglycerides, one of the dangerous fats in the bloodstream. The result of eating too much sugar or drinking too much alcohol is elevated triglyceride levels in the blood. Triglycerides, originating from excess sugar intake, contribute heavily to arteriosclerosis, as does cholesterol, which originates from animal fat.

Let's get back to Harry. Physicians specializing in diabetes refer to the spare tire around his middle as a glucose-meter. Fat accumulating there is predominantly caused by excess sugar (alcohol and carbohydrates). Because fat can dilute insulin, there may not be enough to maintain a normal blood sugar. The result is obesity-onset or type 2 diabetes.

Harry's nightly six-pack represents nine hundred calories of carbohydrates. A pound of fat represents roughly three thousand calories, so Harry's six-pack creates about 1/3 pound of fat.

America's love affair with alcohol is one factor in the obesity epidemic in our culture. It also accounts for a frightening increase in heart disease and hypertension from the elevated triglycerides and type 2 diabetes.

When I quit drinking, I lost eight pounds and one inch from my waistline within several months. I also stopped having very troubling bouts of hypoglycemia or low blood sugar. I used to get shaky and weak an hour or so after eating a doughnut, cookie, or anything with concentrated sugar. The intake of sugar produces an overly brisk release of insulin, which rapidly drops the blood sugar, producing the wobbliness. When the liver is functioning properly, it stores glycogen, which serves as an emergency supply of glucose to prevent attacks of hypoglycemia. When the blood sugar drops from the insulin release, the liver breaks down glycogen into glucose units and releases it into the bloodstream to mitigate the impending hypoglycemia. Alcohol prevents the liver from storing glycogen. Unwittingly, I had been causing my hypoglycemia by drinking.

ALCOHOL, OBESITY, AND DIABETES

WES

My friend Wes told me that, at his worst, he filled a tumbler with vodka, put a straw in it, and set it on his nightstand when he staggered into bed at night. That way, he could get his blood alcohol level back up quickly in the morning to avoid withdrawal.

THE SOBERING TRUTH

26

CIRRHOSIS

The end stage damage of an alcoholic liver is cirrhosis. The term was first used in the 1830s by the famous physician Laennec. It means, in general, a "yellowish scarring or fibrosis", but in medical parlance, it refers to a liver hopelessly scarred from chronic inflammation, most commonly by alcohol. Emphasis on hopeless.

The liver is an organ that has many functions including metabolism and bile production.

The microscopic architecture of the liver is very complex. Hepatocytes or liver cells have the wall of a small blood vessel on one side, and a tiny bile duct on the other. The incoming blood delivers nutrients to the liver cell or hepatocyte, providing raw materials for the cell to use for its many synthetic functions. It also degrades worn out hemoglobin to bilirubin (aka bile) which it secretes into the bile duct.

The functions of the liver are numerous, including metabolism of nutrients, synthesis of lipids, proteins, and fatty acids, and the creation of bile from erythrocytes. The bile is secreted into a bile duct on the opposite side of the cell from its nutrient blood supply.

When multiple hepatocytes are killed due to some toxin such as alcohol, stellate cells in the liver form fibrous tissue to repair the damage. The result of recurrent and massive cell death is massive scarring and some regeneration of hepatocytes, but if the damage is severe and recurrent, the liver cells no longer maintain their delicate microscopic connections with the bile ducts. Bile builds up in the blood, staining the tissues, eyes, and the patient's skin yellow.

The progressive scarring of the liver increases the pressure in the veins there, blood backs up and swells the vessels in the stomach and esophagus, causing varicose veins that have very thin walls that can bleed easily. Many an end-stage alcoholic has ruptured esophageal or gastric varices while vomiting and bled to death into their stomach.

I drank hard in college as did many of my fraternity brothers. I know of at least one who died of end stage liver disease, rupturing esophageal and gastric varices.

27

LESSER-KNOWN HEALTH PROBLEMS DUE TO ALCOHOL

George was back in the hospital again. His temperature was 102.5 degrees Fahrenheit. His eyes watered down his pink, puffy face. Beefy red patches covered his forehead, scalp, and nearly 50 percent of the rest of his body. The remainder was pink and swollen almost to the point of weeping. It was generalized, erythrodermic psoriasis. He was toxic, and he was drunk.

Over many years, physicians have observed that almost every rash is worse if the patient is a heavy drinker. When I worked at the VA hospital during my residency and, subsequently, when I was teaching, I continually observed the high correlation between people with bad psoriasis or eczema and heavy drinking. Long philosophical discussions resulted as we debated the question of whether alcoholics with the genetic predisposition develop psoriasis or whether the stigma of bad psoriasis makes people drunks.

It may be difficult to understand this question if you have never seen severe psoriasis. It causes large, raised pink-to-red scaling patches of skin anywhere on the body. The elbows and knees are generally the worst, but it can affect the entire front of the leg and arm. The scalp is commonly involved, and the process resembles an industrial-strength case of dandruff or cradle cap. The appearance of a person with severe psoriasis may frighten the uninitiated observer. You wouldn't want him sitting next to you on the bus or in the dermatologist's waiting room.

People with psoriasis are very self-conscious about their appearance. Psychological studies have shown they have a very poor self-image, an altered perception of their body. They are also more likely to have depression.

Interestingly, recent scientific studies have shown that an alteration in the immune system cause psoriasis. A subset of T lymphocytes are abnormal, the Th1 lymphocytes. This leads to the abnormal production of messenger chemicals that increase inflammation, producing the pink, scaly skin that we recognize as psoriasis.

Eczema (atopic dermatitis) is a very itchy, scaly skin disease that has an allergic basis. It is commonly associated with hay fever, asthma, food allergies, and a history of other family members who have the same. It is even more common than psoriasis. In its severe form, it is just as physically and socially debilitating. It turns out that an alteration in another subset of T lymphocytes, the Th2 lymphocytes, causes eczema. They produce a completely different group of messenger chemicals, including an antibody called IgE, which is responsible for the release of histamine, the culprit chemical that produces the agonizing itch that is the hallmark of eczema. Have you ever had a horrible itch from poison oak or scabies? People with eczema live with that kind of itch all the time.

So why the lesson in dermatology? Alcohol has been proven to enhance the alteration in both the Th1 and Th2 systems and amplifies inflammation. It aggravates both psoriasis and eczema. And, as these conditions worsen, the psychological stress increases, the drinking increases, and the condition flares to a greater degree, creating a cycle of increasing intensity.

Intake of alcohol greatly increases the abnormal antibody IgE, which causes the allergic symptoms in all three of the allergic triad (eczema, asthma, and hay fever). A bad asthmatic needs to give up his nightly half-liter of wine.

It has long been observed that alcoholics get more infections and more unusual infections than the general population. It was thought that was due to the neglect of personal hygiene, inattention to minor problems before they become major, and abnormal life circumstances that severe chronic alcoholism produces. But it's more than that. I see chronic, intractable infections in successful businessmen who drink a lot. I see fungus infections that are resistant to treatment, and they seem anecdotally to be much more common in alcoholics than in nondrinkers. This occurs because heavy drinkers are immune-suppressed. Their immune systems are not as robust as they would be in an alcohol-free environment.

The hard-drinking, successful businessman will not accept that the itchy pimples on his scalp are due to his heavy drinking. Most people are in denial about their drinking, and they flat-out lie to me about their daily consumption. But they want me to fix them. They don't want to modify any behaviors, especially giving up their two-martini lunches and bottle of wine with dinner. They just want me to make them better. It is an interesting phenomenon. These people are used to being in control and getting what they want. They hold me personally responsible for their disease, and it's my responsibility to cure them. There must be a pill they can take or a salve they can apply. Sadly, it is a theme of much of our society's health woes. We don't want to change our diet or lifestyle. We just want a pill to fix it so we can keep on with the way we want to live. Patients with this mind-set are very hard to treat.

So, if alcohol decreases or alters immune function and immune function is responsible for tumor surveillance, does that mean alcoholics more commonly get cancer? The answer is probably. That study has not been done, but it should be. Certainly, alcoholics get some cancers more commonly. As we discussed previously, mouth, throat, and esophageal cancers are much more common in people with heavy alcohol intake. Smoking and alcohol seem to be cofactors in all three of those diseases, but alcohol alone may serve to promote them in a number of people. Liver, colon, and breast cancers are known to be increased in people who drink alcohol. There is an increased probability that pancreatic cancer is also caused by alcohol intake, though the hard data is, as yet, unavailable. But in addition to the cancers known to be caused by alcohol, a generalized predisposition to all kinds of cancer may be brought about by the decrease in the vitality of the immune system hindered by chronic alcohol intake. And, as stated earlier, once cancer is present in the body, regular alcohol intake may promote its spread.

For the middle-aged woman, alcohol may aggravate many of the symptoms of menopause, especially the generalized dilation of blood vessels known as hot flashes. The mechanism is simply the additive effect of dilation of blood vessels brought on by alcohol.

Considering the many negative health effects of alcohol, I am amazed that anyone would drink. Of course, many drinkers are unaware of the facts because they have not been well publicized. Hopefully, this book will serve that end and help to counter the barrage of alcohol lobby-generated press releases concerning the beneficial effects of alcohol. Then, well-informed people can choose to drink or not based on a full understanding of alcohol's benefits and risks.

JIM WELLS

I received an e-mail from an old college buddy last night. He reported that Jim Wells died last week of alcoholic liver failure. A brilliant athlete and all-American volleyball player, Jim was one of the best setters in the game. He was a year ahead of me in school. A little blond-haired surfer dude, he had grown up playing beach volleyball in Manhattan Beach. No telling when he had started drinking.

28

FETAL ALCOHOL SYNDROME

In labor for twelve hours and hard labor for the last two, Stacey was exhausted. But she was young and strong, and she desperately wanted this child. Stacey and Tom were ecstatic about the prospect of their firstborn. They had been married five years. They were established financially, and they had traveled. As Stacey put it, they had "done the self-indulgent, selfish things" so neither would resent the financial demand and time restraints of a new baby. Stacey took a leave of absence from her work as human resources director for the local community college. Tom's insurance business was thriving and could offset Stacey's loss of income.

Another contraction increased in intensity. Stacey gripped the rails of the table, her contorted face revealing the effort.

"There's a head, Stacey. Keep pushing!"

Dr. Johnson's skilled hands gently turned the head, sweeping the mouth and throat with a finger to clear it of debris, and delivered the shoulders, torso, and, finally, tiny hands and feet. He was so focused on the task that he hadn't noticed the child as yet. He held the infant by the legs, spanked him on the buttocks to produce a hoarse cry, and then placed the baby on Stacey's belly.

"Here's your healthy—" He noticed the face. He said nothing. The silence was deafening.

"What's wrong, doctor?" Stacey knew something was. Terror welled up within her.

Dr. Johnson silently stared. The facial features were unmistakable. The tiny face was flattened centrally, looking as if it had been pressed against a plate glass window. The cheeks had almost no curve to them. The upper lip was thin without the delicate upward curve of Cupid's bow. The eyes were abnormally small, set wide apart, and appeared sunken into the face. He dreaded times like these. It had happened only twenty-five or so times in his career, but there was no easy way to handle it. Rousing from his silence, the professional of thirty years took over.

"This little guy seems to have some problems."

Stacey fought back hysteria. "What is it, doctor?" She sobbed, exhausted physically and emotionally.

"Stacey, do you drink much?"

Her prenatal history form revealed no alcohol intake, but Dr. Johnson knew that information was not always reliable.

"Only on weekends, and not that much then."

"Were you ever drunk during your pregnancy?"

"I had a glass of wine on the weekend with friends, but never---"

She suddenly remembered. There had been the week with friends on a houseboat at Lake Powell. It was before she knew she was pregnant. They had drunk quite a bit. Her long silence accented the tomblike atmosphere of the delivery room.

"Well, I am no expert, Stacey, but I am concerned that this little guy may have some physical changes due to alcohol. We'll call Dr. Patterson to get his input. I'm sorry."

Dr. Albert Patterson, a noted expert in newborn syndromes who taught at the university medical school, confirmed the diagnosis. Baby Boy Griffith suffered from fetal alcohol syndrome (FAS). For parents Tom and Stacey, a life of grief, disappointment, and hard work was about to begin.

Dustin Griffith was a floppy baby, a term given to infants with decreased muscle tone, which would later be reflected in poor muscle coordination. His congenital neurological defects, brought on by alcohol in his mother's circulation while critical areas of his brain and nervous system were developing, would make him a lifelong challenge for his parents and society. He would have a low IQ, poor memory, poor anger management, low academic ability, poor impulse control, and a severe form of attention deficit disorder. He would require special schooling all through his formative years, and only with extreme good fortune would he be able to be a productive member of society, working at a minimum wage job.

Most people think FAS occurs only in mothers who are hard-core alcoholics. That isn't so. Although it is true that severe FAS occurs in babies born to chronic alcoholics, growth retardation and fetal neurological deficits may be produced by maternal intake of as little as one drink (one-and-a-half ounces of alcohol, five ounces of wine, and twelve ounces of beer) a day. It has also been associated with heavy episodic drinking, like Stacey's party at the lake.

The effects are devastating. FAS and the more subtle alcohol-related neurodevelopmental disorders (ARND) are the tragic and shameful secrets of a society that does not recognize that alcohol is a real health hazard. First described in 1968 by Lemoine in France, FAS has been the subject of intense research during the last decade (Miller). That first description is likened to discovering the tip of the iceberg. For every child with clinically apparent FAS,[10] there are many more children with learning disabilities, behavior problems, hyperactivity, and attention deficit directly related to maternal alcohol use (Mayoch).

How does this happen? It is important to remember that alcohol is a cell poison. Its metabolism produces chemicals called free radicals that can cause mutations, death of, or damage to cells. Of all developing organs in the human body, the brain is the most vulnerable to this damage.

Alcohol inhibits the production of cholesterol in the brain (Gundogan). Given our negative impression of cholesterol, that sounds like a good thing, but cholesterol is critical to the developing brain (Merrick). It is used to create cell membranes of nerve cells and synapses between nerve cells (Burd). A certain level is necessary for nerve cell survival. Without it, nerve cells do not develop. The critical and elaborate connections, the synapses, are not produced (Gundogan).

Alcohol readily crosses the placenta into the fetal circulation, so the fetus is exposed to the same blood alcohol level as the mother (Fryer).

---

[10] *The estimate is close to 1 percent of all births.*

Alcohol produces injury in all three trimesters of pregnancy. The resultant damage depends on what part of the body, particularly the brain, is developing at the time of intoxication.

In the first trimester, the neurons and their supporting structural cells and blood vessels are organizing and migrating into primitive centers that will later be discrete areas of the brain, specifically brain stem, cerebellum, and cerebrum (27). This is done by a part of the fetal brain called the organizer that is extremely dependent on a form of vitamin A (retinoic acid). By inhibiting retinoic acid, alcohol produces gross deformities in the way the brain is organized (McGee).

Alcohol also has a profound effect on the placenta, the lifeline organ that supplies the developing fetus with oxygen and nutrients. Alcohol exposure results in growth retardation of the placenta (Gemma). It is no wonder that first trimester alcohol exposure may produce small birth weight, small head (microcephaly), and small brain size (Pragst).

The second trimester accounts for more of the advanced organization and development of the brain. Not surprisingly, alcohol exposure during this period produces more clinically relevant features of FAS. The cerebellum is responsible for muscle coordination and balance. Damage to Purkinje nerve cells in the cerebellum impairs these functions (J. et al.)

The cerebral cortex is the thinking and feeling part of the brain. Impaired development and organization here produces learning disabilities and behavioral problems seen later in these individuals.

The hypothalamus is a tiny area on the undersurface on the brain that is vital to monitoring and regulating our internal environment (temperature, blood pressure, and so forth). The hypothalamus communicates with the adjacent pituitary gland that produces hormones that regulate many of the endocrine glands, particularly the adrenal gland, the body's best responder to stress. Prenatal alcohol exposure permanently creates an overstimulation of the hypothalamus-pituitary-adrenal mechanism. The result is the body feeling chronically stressed. FAS individuals have more illnesses throughout life as a consequence (Fryer).

During and after the second trimester, alcohol has a profound effect on blood flow to the fetal brain (Li). Normally, when oxygen is decreased in the fetal brain, there is a reflex increase in blood flow to compensate.

This reflex is suppressed after alcohol exposure, making the fetus more susceptible to brain damage in the last trimester and during labor and delivery when pressure on the head passing through the birth canal may decrease cerebral blood flow (Li).

In the final trimester, the brain is developing widespread connections that integrate information, form memory, control motor activities, and allow complex problem-solving. These and many brain tasks, termed executive functions, are accomplished in the frontal lobes of the cerebrum, notably the prefrontal cortex. This area is profoundly affected developmentally with maternal alcohol intake (Calhoun).

A small area at the base of the cerebrum is called the hippocampus because it is shaped like a horse. Neuronal development here is associated with mood, learning, and memory, especially math and reading abilities (29). Alcohol disturbs the development of the hippocampus in all three trimesters of pregnancy and even after birth (Jiang).

Finally, and perhaps the most frightening of all, there is strong evidence that alcohol exposure in gestation sensitizes the developing brain, making the individual more susceptible to alcoholism as an adult (Shankar).

Currently, FAS is not treatable. Studies in laboratory animals show treatment with aniracetam in the first few days of extra-uterine life may partially ameliorate the effects (Ieraci). Early diagnosis then becomes critical. That can be accomplished by testing newborn hair and/or meconium for fatty acid ethyl esters (FAEE) and ethylglucoronide, both of which are increased in FAS (Chee). Given the magnitude of the public health problem that FAS presents, it seems vital to do this, but mandatory testing may be viewed as a violation of personal rights and raise a public outcry.

Whatever the outcome of that debate, it seems critical to make an effort to prevent FAS. The public needs to know the risk of drinking during pregnancy. As little as one-half ounce of alcohol daily can lower a child's IQ. There is probably no safe minimum of alcohol for the pregnant woman.

The American Academy of Pediatrics recommends a program of public education at the high school and college level to make young women aware that there is no safe amount of alcohol that can be consumed immediately before or during pregnancy. Complete abstinence from alcohol in women who are pregnant or are planning to get pregnant is the only sure prevention.

29

MY LIFE WITH THE BOTTLE: *PART II*

I carried a lot of emotional baggage as I made the transition from college to medical school. I had my amphetamine addiction, an uncertainty I could handle the workload after four years of poor study habits, and a broken heart from a failed first serious relationship. From the start, I was in trouble. I went to class, but just couldn't study at night. It was the educational equivalent of writer's block. But I had my supply of Eskatrol. My dental school chum had hooked me up with his doctor. Likewise, I had been put on Dr. Wayne Callings' weight loss program, which included, of course, a prescription for Eskatrol.

Transitioning from undergraduate to medical school was a shock. I attended class eight hours a day, five days a week. I'd arrive home exhausted and stare at textbooks the size of telephone books, the language of which I couldn't begin to understand. When I tried to read one, I had to look up every third word in a medical dictionary. I was terrified. Like a deer in the headlights, I was paralyzed. Midterms rolled around, and I pulled three all-nighters with my trusty Eskatrol. I learned the entire anatomy of the head and neck in one night. When I walked into the exam the next morning, I felt confident. But as I read each question, it seemed that at least two answers of the five multiples were correct.

Which one was more correct?

I skipped to the next question, only to find the same scenario. When

I finished the exam, I had answered only eighteen of the sixty questions. Panic began to creep in as I went back through, trying to divine which of the two correct answers was more correct. I looked at my watch. Only ten minutes was left. The faster I tried to go, the more panicked I became. Finally, the bell rang. I had left ten questions unanswered. I bombed the exam, barely making a passing grade.

That anatomy exam set the tone for the entire year. I was so fearful of studying that I couldn't, and I didn't. I crammed in a hyperintense atmosphere and then choked on the exams. School, my personal life, and the speed combined to create a nightmare of fear and dread. I finished the year sixtieth in a class of sixty-four. I was miserable. The worst aspect of my dependence on Eskatrol was coming down from four days straight on the drug. There was a rebound of exhaustion and depression that was almost unbearable, coupled with physical pain as the drug cleared my system.

I was not the only drug user in the freshman class. Half my classmates were taking speed to study. Most fared better than I did. Several did not. One unlucky classmate, a pharmacological adventurer who shared a cadaver with me in anatomy, fried his brain on the last day of finals and wrote an entire ten-page blue book, ironically on psychiatric disorders, on the first page of the book, writing each page over the preceding one. The page was illegible, and he failed the exam, that class, and several others. He was asked to repeat the year. He did and now prospers as a psychiatrist somewhere in the affluence and neuroses of southern California.

The end of my freshman year brought an honest appraisal and reevaluation of the direction my life had taken. I knew I could not continue my chemical roller coaster. I wouldn't survive. I had the summer to find an exit strategy. By some miracle, I learned of a summer research fellowship in neurosurgery with a world-renowned doctor in the field, and I was accepted. Unknowingly, I was about to forge a relationship that would change my life. Robert H. Pudenz, MD, who had recently lost his son to suicide, would heal my wounds of fear and self-doubt as I healed his profound grief. Dr. Pudenz believed in me completely and taught me to believe in myself. The work I did with him that and the following summer was some of the finest I have ever done. I began the new academic year resolved I would never take drugs to study, even if it meant failing out. I was good to my word. I earned straight As that second year and went from sixtieth to sixteenth in my class. My life was completely turned around. I recognized I had been addicted to speed and I had some characteristics of an addictive personality. Sadly, I didn't recognize I had the same problem with alcohol, only a less severe, less obvious, and seemingly more harmless one. I didn't drink any more than most of my friends did, certainly a lot less than my parents and a lot less than I had in the fraternity. But alcohol was an intimate friend, something I enjoyed, looked forward to, and needed. I might have been a long way upstream, but I was in the current, headed for the rapids above a deadly waterfall. It would take thirty years to get to the brink and the necessity to swim for my life. Thank God I made it. How unfortunate that I couldn't learn the lesson when I was in medical school.

You may be thinking, "He's overreacting. He didn't really have a problem. He functioned well. Maybe he needed a drink now and then to relax or unwind, but he wasn't an alcoholic."

That may be true for some people, but it wasn't true for me. I now know that I drank alcohol for the chemical effect it had on me, just as I took Eskatrol to study. I was developing a physiological and social need for alcohol, although it was barely recognizable for many years. But that's the way alcohol is. You drink it seemingly harmlessly for many years. Then, one day, if you are lucky, you wake up to the fact that it has changed you. It changed me. I was a different person when I drank. It changed my personality. I was more skeptical, cynical, mistrusting, angry, and, at times, downright mean. And after many years, I realized alcohol could really make me depressed. I was using alcohol out of habit, but also because I thought it helped me cope with anxiety, stress, and depression. It doesn't. It is a poor drug for all three, and it can increase depression as it did for me. I finally quit because I didn't like the person I was when I drank. I didn't like what my friends became when they drank. Now my feelings and the person I am are both real. I am not altered by alcohol. And I genuinely like myself sober a lot more.

Another of my addictive behaviors was smoking. I began the day I moved into the dorms my freshman year of college and continued through the middle of my second year of medical school. I was really something, pulling those allnighters my first year in med school, drinking Diet Coke or coffee, puffing away on a cigarette, and reading a textbook. The second quarter of my freshman year, I smoked so heavily the last night of finals that I burned the roof of my mouth. It sloughed out in one thick, leathery piece two days later. I was subconsciously disgusted, but laughed about it to all my friends. I considered it a necessary evil to help me get through school.

In the second quarter of my sophomore year in med school, after I had successfully given up speed, I did my very first physical examination on a patient as a student doctor. The patient was dying of end-stage emphysema, and I was shocked at the cruelty of that disease. He had been a steelworker, helping to build some of the high-rise buildings that dotted the Los Angeles skyline. In his prime, he was two hundred and thirty pounds, standing six-foot-two. He weighed one hundred and sixteen pounds when I examined him, a skin-covered skeleton. He panted like a wheezing steam engine, trying to deliver precious oxygen to lungs that couldn't absorb it. He was so short of breath that he couldn't close his mouth to chew a bite of food, and he could only answer my questions in monosyllables.

I had never seen emphysema up close. After several prior failed attempts to quit smoking, I took an intimate look at the ravages of this disease and never smoked again. This was the third example of the addictive nature of my personality, but I never connected my prior addictions to speed and tobacco with my use of alcohol. I saw myself as a social drinker, like all my friends, and certainly no more than that. It was the norm to drink on the weekends and at parties, and it was okay to get a little tipsy on occasion. It is fascinating to reflect back now that I didn't know any nondrinkers. No one was around to question the premise. There was nothing to alter the behavior and nothing to challenge the denial.

In medical school and in residency, my finances and social status allowed me to begin to drink hard liquor. The beer and cheap wine gave way to distilled spirits and good wine. I tried gin and tonics, vodka and tonics, and bourbon and seven, and I settled on scotch and water. My wife and I took some wine-tasting classes and joined a club with several other residents in my training program. We read books, sampled, and began to develop a taste for fine wines. Well on the way to becoming wine snobs, we bought some good wine to put away and rented a locker at a local liquor store that was temperature and humidity controlled to store our considerable investment.

I quit the hard stuff after Joe got me sick on it. Several years into my residency, it came about as the result of a dinner at my in-laws' house. Joe, my father-in-law, was the quintessential salesman, possessing a toothy smile and a hearty handshake. We dined with them one evening after I had spent several consecutive near all-nighters staffing an emergency room. I was fuzzy with fatigue, and his scotch tasted good. Joe was not one to skimp on the alcohol, and he made sure my glass was refilled promptly. After three or four scotch and waters that were mostly scotch, I was pretty drunk. My wife drove home. I was very sick, but, borrowing a page from my college days, I unloaded as much of the dinner and alcohol as I could as soon as we got home. From a very early age, I've excelled at self-induced vomiting. As a kid, I developed horrendous headaches from eating pork. Eventually, it would make me vomit. As soon as I did, my headache disappeared. As a result, I learned to gag myself with my finger and induce retching. It came in handy during my college years, and it helped that night when Joe plied me with scotch. Despite relieving myself of probably half the scotch, I still felt awful the next day. I made my wife promise she wouldn't let on to her dad. I felt bad enough and didn't want to give Joe the satisfaction of knowing how ill I had been. After that, I lost my taste for scotch and gave up other distilled spirits. The alcohol content was too high. It was possible to drink too much too fast and get way beyond a controllable level of intoxication. I would drink wine with meals and a margarita or fancy rum concoction on occasion, but, as time went on, I became almost exclusively a beer drinker. I love the taste of beer. With its relatively low alcohol content, I could drink quite a bit without getting drunk. And if I did start feeling drunk, I could ease up and control the level of intoxication much more easily than I could when drinking hard liquor. I never rationalized that I wasn't drinking that much. I knew and agreed with the old adage, "If you drink a lot of beer, you drink a lot." But it was a more user-friendly vehicle that fit my lifestyle, and I liked the taste.

After I quit smoking, I took up another addiction. I began to run. Running is more than an activity that produces fitness. It is a passion that can become an addiction. I was aware of that at some level, but I rationalized it was a healthy addiction. I ran out of resolve to control a lifelong weight problem and mitigate the stress of medical school and the emotional intensity that studying produced. After three or four hours of studying, usually with several cups of coffee, an hour long run would relax me, allow my racing mind to slow down, and permit precious sleep.

I ran for five years on my own for exercise and fitness and as a stress-releaser. I began with a mile a day and then three. After five years, I was running six miles a day with an occasional ten-mile run on the weekend. Then one day, another runner pulled up on my shoulder, complimented my pace, and invited me to his running club's half-marathon the next day. I didn't think much of my ability, and the idea of running against others in competition intimidated me. But curiosity got the better of me, and I showed up the next day and ran the half-marathon (13.1 miles) in eighty-one minutes. That finished me well up in the pack and earned the congratulations of many of the club's runners. Realizing my time was well under the pace required to achieve the sub-three-hour qualification to run the Boston Marathon, I was hooked. I made the abrupt transition from recreational runner to serious running junkie.

Running and beer drinking are practically synonymous. The beverage of choice after a long, hot training run is an ice-cold lager or two or five. I used to joke that running was an excuse to drink beer, and it was partially true. Some of the best fellowship I have ever experienced was sitting on the lawn after a hard run and drinking a six-pack or two with a bunch of running buddies. There was camaraderie and a commonness of purpose that was intimate and very satisfying. Runners are a great group. Intensely fit, they value physical effort and discipline. Unlike my often-arrogant physician acquaintances, they come from every walk of life. I was good enough, just barely, to be one of them. Within this circle, there was a broad spectrum of running abilities from college cross-country medalists to fitness runners. An amiable and gregarious group, they all shared the love of running and beer.

Running fulfilled a great many of my needs. I had always struggled

MY LIFE WITH THE BOTTLE: PART II

with a weight problem, and running allowed me to control it. When I first started in the early 1970s, I developed a running variant of anorexia nervosa. During my quarter of med school in England, I went more than a little bit overboard on the running. British school didn't start until nine o'clock in the morning, so I ran ten miles each morning before school. I ate only one meal a day, dinner, and I controlled my hunger the rest of the time by eating fresh carrots. I'm just shy of six-foot-two. In my chubby days early in med school, I weighed just over two hundred pounds. When I came back from England, I weighed one hundred and fifty-eight pounds. I looked a bit gaunt, and I had an orange cast to my skin from all the beta-carotene.[11] It took a year for me to recover from the anorexia, correct my skewed perception of my body image, and fill out a little. But running, at the level I chose to do it, always allowed me to eat and drink anything I wanted without getting back to my pre-running weight.

Running also gave me a lot of confidence. The discipline required generalized into other areas of my life. I was never as focused and happy as when I was training for a marathon or other big race.

I also experienced the running high a lot. When I was really fit, I felt an intense sense of well-being almost every day. Running is one of nature's antidepressants. The only downside was that I could drink as much as I wanted and not get fat or feel the depression that occurs when people drink heavily. So insight and awareness of the negative effects of alcohol would wait a time when I couldn't continue running.

I ran hard for thirty years. I averaged between fifty and seventy miles a week. Through it all, beer was my training partner. Only once did we part company. In the late 1980s, I was training for a hundred-mile run. As part of my Spartan discipline, I gave up alcohol for the last two months before the race. I remember feeling intensely well, but I thought it was my physical shape. After finishing the race, I drank a quart of Budweiser, savoring the taste. Later, I wistfully wished I had continued my sobriety, but it was too late. I was drinking again.

One of the problems with my personality, physical needs, and chemical makeup is that I can't just drink one beer. I begin to feel that mellowness,

---

[11] It's a very good internal sunscreen and free radical quencher, but that's another story.

and I want another and another. For me, it's all or nothing. So now for me, it's nothing.

If my knees hadn't begun to wear out, I may never have developed the insight I needed to quit drinking. After five arthroscopic surgeries, I finally had to accept the inevitability that I couldn't run at my previous level of intensity. Gone were the endorphin high and the antidepressant. But the beer kept flowing. The result was a bulging middle and a hard-to-pinpoint depression that I attributed to not being able to run, reaching middle age, and stresses of an intensely busy medical practice. It took a long while for me to realize it was the alcohol.

But today, nine years into sobriety, the depression is gone. It is wonderful to know that the feelings I experience are real and not induced by a chemical I've ingested. I have defeated four addictive behaviors in my fifty-plus years: nail biting, smoking, amphetamines, and alcohol. Alcohol was definitely the hardest. The crux of the problem was denial because:

- I had been raised in a family of HFAs and didn't know what normal was.
- I had never missed a day of school or work because of my drinking, which I thought was an important criterion for a problem drinker.
- I had seen real alcoholics in the admitting ward at county hospital, and I was nothing like those people.
- All my friends drank as much or more than I did. I had no point of reference for nondrinking.
- The addictive personality that had trouble with speed and tobacco would not have trouble with alcohol.

30

SARAH'S STORY
GUEST AUTHOR

I hear his footsteps outside in the driveway and breathe in sharply. I hadn't heard him pull up. This time of night, I always tried to be in bed before he got home so I didn't have to interact with him.

I quickly glance at myself in the mirror: sleep shirt, same face, same hair. And yet, a fleeting moment of un-recognition: who was this cold, resentful person? How had she settled in my body, my heart? Her eyes are ice.

The front door of our home quietly opens. I dart out of the bathroom into the small hallway that connects to our kitchen, hoping to make it to bed before he sees me. But here he is, in the tiny hallway now, with me. I'm making my body as small as I can, clinging to the hallway wall so I wouldn't have to be any closer to him. I slightly turn my head away, holding my breath, tensing my body. Please, God, no, I plead inside. Don't make me be here. I can't bear it.

"Sarah," he says softly. I turn to look at him. He's standing in the corner of the hallway. He suddenly looks small to me.

"What," I impatiently mutter back. I want to be anywhere but here—next to him, in this house, in this life. I look down at the floor. I feel anger pounding in my ears.

"I went to this meeting tonight, and everything they said… that was me. And you're right. I am an alcoholic. And I know I've messed a lot of things up and caused you a lot of pain, but I'm going to do everything I can to make it better. I promise. And I'm sorry."

For a flash of a moment, like the brief pause between inhaling and exhaling where that small yet spacious calm resides, I feel a spark. This is different. He's never referred to himself as an alcoholic before. I look up at his face briefly, and the transient moment passes. The anger descends upon me again like a blooming stain. I can feel it curl my lips to a snarl.

"Whatever," I spat back. I turn my back to him and walk quickly away, leaving him in the hallway alone. I'm glad to walk away from him, but even more so, I'm glad to be alone. I make my way back to our dark bedroom where we don't sleep together anymore. The sheets are cold, I am cold and nothing can warm me up.

I can't count the number of times I've heard him say I'm sorry and I'm going to change. The times I believed him, the times I pretended I believed him, the times I lied to myself that I believed him. I wanted so badly to believe him. But drinking always won that game.

I kept playing the game, though. It's a lonely, devastating game where no one wins. Feeling alone right next to someone is one of the saddest places to be, I found. I always hated falling asleep feeling the warmth of his body next to me, but he was a million miles away, passed out in a drunken stupor. I'd lie on my back and cry hot, silent tears that would weave their way down my cheeks and fall wet on my pillow.

It was a painful dichotomy to be enduring a life with an alcoholic while simultaneously carrying on with an existence that looked "normal" from the outside. When I dropped off our oldest child at school, I would think, "no one else is going through this", and the shame would envelop me. I wanted to be normal. I wasn't.

Eventually the pain hardened to anger. And I had searing anger. For every beer can I picked up, for every drop of piss I cleaned off the bathroom floor, for all the empty bottles of booze I found in his sock drawer that I counted, for every window curtain I put back up that he had tried to hold his balance with, for the neglect I shouldered time and time and time again, for his inability to be the father I had hoped my children would have, for the dream I had for my life that was shot down.

The anger solidified for me in a precise moment. The moment I sealed my heart shut from him. Becoming impenetrable to him was my greatest protector.

I was standing in our small kitchen carrying a birthday cake I made for our oldest child. The lights are dimmed and the candles are lit and I'm singing happy birthday,

"Happy birthday to you…! Blow the candles out! Make a wish!" I sing to him. He is so little and so excited. The glow of the candles illuminates both his and his younger sister's face. I happen to look up right before he blows the candles out to see my husband. He is standing there, swaying back and forth, drunk with his eyes heavy and glazed over. Smoking pot, drinking—I don't have to smell his breath to check or search for bottles or ask where he has been anymore—I know. There is no question.

"He doesn't belong here," I think. As he stands there swaying in the dim radiance of our son's birthday candles, time slows down for me. In a very fixed and quiet way, a decision, like an axe blade making a clean cut, was made inside me as I looked across the table at him.

"I hate you," I thought, straightforwardly and simply. That was it. Like a silent squall. No sound to the wreckage. Screaming underwater. Swallowing pain until it seeps sick into your soul. Awful and soundless, yet precise and exacting.

"You're raising your children with an alcoholic father, Sarah, and it's not ok." These words a trusted friend said hit me low and deep and I turned them over in my head for days and days. I knew it wasn't ok. And I knew what I had to do.

My heart had vacated our relationship a long time ago, but I was afraid to ask him to leave. I didn't know how I would explain it to our children. I thought of their young, confused hearts and what their faces would look like when I told them. I thought of being a single mom. I thought about the small, everyday things that would be different; like changing the light bulbs at the height of our kitchen, not having someone to open jars that I couldn't, how to fix or build… anything. It was all of these things, some seemingly small, that gave me pause, that filled me with grief. These seemingly small realities were really evidence of a life and dream falling apart.

I used to go out to the bluffs not far from where we lived and look out at the endless ocean. It took me out of myself to see that powerful ebbing and flowing. To see the world going on as it does, despite the fact that my inner world was crumbling.

"What do you want me to do, God?" I would speak out to the grey sky and grey waters. "Tell me," I would plead. I never heard anything. But I'd stand there waiting, until I was too cold. Then I'd wipe my tears, get back in the car and drive home.

The night my husband met me in the hallway and told me he was an alcoholic was right after I decided to ask him to leave. I would do it this week, I decided. I had been building up courage. I didn't know he was at a meeting for alcoholics that night. I didn't know his sobriety had begun.

I had always thought that when he stopped drinking, everything would be fixed. Things got harder in a new way when he stopped drinking.

The damage to our relationship was great, and my anger even greater. I had built an island that I only allowed myself and our two children to inhabit. I had built a life away from him that was protective. When I had shared with a friend before his sobriety began that I was afraid of being a single mom, he looked at me and said, "You already are a single mom." That stopped my in my tracks. I had gotten used to functioning alone.

I resisted letting him in at all costs. I wanted to leave the relationship. I was drowning in bitterness, pain and grief and I didn't know how to let him in. And I didn't want to.

After the first support group I attended for people with loved ones who were alcoholics, I took all the literature and pamphlets and threw them in the trash. I kept the doors to my heart firmly shut.

I wandered in and out of my days, a busy young mom, boiling underneath my daily tasks with resentment and a deep wish for a different life. Despite his sobriety, a despairing discontent and unhappiness raged constantly inside me.

At the brink of separating from my husband, I left to go spend a few days alone in Ojai, a small town in southern California. I went on hikes and took myself out to eat and moved my body in yoga classes. I felt momentarily free, away from the angst that filled our home. But I still didn't understand why, now that my husband was sober, I didn't want to be with him. I wanted to love my husband, but I didn't. I didn't want to go home. I cried in the car as I drove back.

Upon my return, it was my husband who encouraged me to attend another support meeting. I begrudgingly went.

It was in a large room with chairs pushed together facing a common wall where a wooden podium stood. There was a shelf in the back corner with books to purchase with titles like "Paths to Recovery" and "Courage to Change". The book titles made me cringe with confusion and anger. Why did I have to go to a meeting when he was the one with the problem? I didn't have a problem, he did.

The meeting began, and I was welcomed as a newcomer, my voice sounding small as I introduced myself. As I sat in this circle with people of all ages and genders, I listened. I listened to their stories about their sisters or wives or friends or fathers whose alcoholism scarred their lives, from the past or currently. I was stunned with shock and simultaneously felt connected as I listened to their stories. I felt for the first time that I wasn't alone. I believe this was the first brush I had with healing— knowing I wasn't alone.

What began unraveling me further was when I heard these people talk about tending to themselves, instead of the alcoholic. They spoke of the effort it took to try to control the addict. I had never viewed my actions as ones of control. It stunned me to see that's exactly what they were. I had thought I was helping. They spoke of having boundaries, of saying no when they needed to, of considering their own lives and needs. When they weren't doing that, and instead were trying to manage the alcoholic, they considered themselves as sick.

In that meeting, I learned I was doing every single thing that was recommended not to do as someone who was involved with an alcoholic. It was extremely humbling, and I felt myself stagger inside with the breath sucking realization that I was not well. All those years of resentment I had created myself. No one asked me to stay, or clean up after him, or count his drinks or search his phone to find clues as to where he had been. No one had required that I neglect myself—that was all me. I was the one who had given my power over to alcoholism, without ever taking a drink. I felt like I had been plunged in icy cold water, trying to get a breath, shocked. This was an introduction of a completely new way of seeing for me, and it was life altering.

I kept going to that weekly Monday meeting and started learning new ways to do things, and how to care for myself. I became more familiar with the people there and their lives. I felt cared for when they would check in on me at the meetings, simply asking how everything was going with an understanding look in their eyes. It was like a balm to my restless spirit. I also heard the same sayings each time like "one day at a time" and "take it easy", which only weeks before that initial meeting would have completely baffled me. How on earth could I "take it easy" when I wanted to rip the walls down and scream? But the more I shared, the more I felt seen, and the more I felt seen, the more alive I seemed to come. This was healing in motion.

One Monday meeting stands out to me in particular. It was my turn to share in the circle on that week's topic. I took a breath to make sure that was I was saying came from a place of truth, and not from what I thought I should say or what I thought others wanted to hear. Honesty with myself and others was a grueling lesson I was learning.

I don't remember exactly what I shared that day, only that I felt calm and rooted in myself. Part of the way through my share, to my far left, a large brunette woman at least 10 years my senior, raised her hands towards the ceiling while hollering,

"Girl! Speak that truth! Keep talking! Mmm that's good! I feel you girl!" I paused, shocked. People around the room laughed. In that moment, I felt a layer of stone crumble away from my heart. Something left me in that sharing of her affirmation, sending waves of healing through my entire being. She saw me. I wanted to crawl onto her great lap and weep.

When it was her turn to share, the grit and grueling pain of her story practically brought me to my knees. Tears welled up in my eyes as she spoke.

It was the people in that room that helped me feel like I wasn't alone, that understood my journey even if our stories were different, that supported me with their own experiences of hope and pain. And in the raw humanity of that shared hope and pain, my heart began to thaw. Slowly.

My husband was sober and it was like becoming acquainted all over again. My anger still smoldered and the hurt ran deep, but in small moments, I started letting him near me. Perhaps laughing at a joke together, maybe thanking him for something he did for me.

I remember beginning to ask him questions about his life from before we met and into the early days of our relationship, which began when we were both 19. I began to feel a curiosity about this man, my husband, that I hadn't before. I still recoiled at his touch, but I remember physically feeling something beginning to melt inside me as we spoke more and I learned more about him. This something started melting until it felt like a torrent, ripping my heart open.

I wanted the torrent to stop. I didn't want to love him, and I was angry with myself that I did. I didn't want to forgive him. I wanted to punish him. But my heart was beating raw and wild, and denying it sucked the life force out of me. I was angry with God, "Please don't let me love him," I would plead through streams of tears.

He began coming on my hikes simply because he wanted to. This caught me by surprise and I searched for reasons why he would be lying about wanting to spend time with me. I questioned that there wasn't somewhere else he actually wanted to be. But he was there, with me, by choice, climbing a dusty mountain trail. We started having deep conversations on those hikes, talking like we never had before. This was connection, something I had been dying for, and it moved me greatly. It was deeply nourishing for me, and for him too.

Building trust takes time, however. I had a hard time accepting this new reality of him being sober and wanting to spend time with our family. I was always looking for a reason why he would leave for something "better".

One day, he walked out of the house to get something out of his car. I had a flash in my mind of a time I had found an empty wine bottle in his car. Before I even knew what I was doing, I was racing out the door and flying down the porch steps. I was convinced he was getting booze he had hidden in his car. As I ran wildly down the driveway towards his car, he heard me and looked up. I stopped in the middle of the driveway. The trunk of his car was open and he had a pack of soda water in his hands. He stood there, staring at me, and I at him. We were silent, frozen in a present moment that was clouded with the past. We both knew why I ran out there. I felt embarrassed as I turned around and walked back inside. Trust takes time.

He attended many meetings to support his sobriety, and I was surprised at how hard it was for me. I felt selfish. Drinking had taken him away from our family, now becoming sober does too? When he was at meetings, I imagined he was out drinking somewhere with buddies, creating a whole narrative that would have me reeling by the time he got home. Only to hear, when he arrived, about his zeal and enthusiasm he was finding in sobriety. I still had healing to do.

He made new connections and friends and his life expanded considerably. He was doing great, which I was glad for, yet somehow it was hurtful. Once again, I felt selfish. How did he get to romp around drinking for years, messing up lives—now to be having a blast as he discovered sobriety?

I was still crazed from years of centering my entire life on him and his drinking. I felt ashamed and weak and deeply disappointed with myself. It was a hard truth for me to come up against—that I had deserted myself for him and for a life that chipped away at my very soul. I had missed out on opportunities and experiences because I was so caught up in his world. The deepness of that grief shook me to my core.

It was also extremely humbling to see that I had gotten very good at blaming him for anything that was going wrong in my life. I wanted it to be his fault that I was unhappy, and he was easy to blame, but the truth was that I had always had a choice. It was not my fault that he was an alcoholic, but I had chosen to stay again and again in situations that hurt me. It was all my choice. A crumbling and empowering realization, I saw my part in the dance.

I shed old layers of myself bit by bit as truths that were hard to face bubbled up. Therapy helped me. Reading helped me (thank you *Codependent No More* by Melody Beattie!), speaking openly to trusted friends helped me. Rediscovering a Higher Power that supported me helped me. Learning to pray helped me.

I signed up for a local herbal medicine course, something I had always wanted to do. I started working again part time as a massage therapist, which I had put aside for the years of young child rearing. It felt good to help people and get paid for it and my own earnings made me proud. I began hiking more frequently and going to the library simply for the pleasure of it. Small things like joining the local natural foods co-op, my favorite place to shop, felt like a reclamation. Little expressions of living in a way that matched who I was on the inside began to breathe life into me. My friendships deepened as I was honest about my life for the first time, not just about the journey of being married to an alcoholic, but of my dreams and hopes. Even just stating things I liked bolstered my sense of self.

When Winter rolled around, my husband began planning for his annual ski trip with a group of his buddies. I felt the familiar gut tearing panic begin to rear its head. Sometimes, it is so encompassing and intense I have to sit down. And that is what I did after I put the kids to bed that night. I sat on the kitchen floor and pulled my knees into my chest, resting my head on them. I hadn't felt like this for a long time. The tears and panic and anger were so familiar, they almost felt good because I knew them so well. Here I was, reverting to the way I had always done things in the past. But I knew I didn't want to do this anymore. I didn't want to be jerked around by my fear. "God, help me," I breathed into my knees. The more I breathed into the burning pit in my stomach, the more I was able to calm down.

What am I afraid of? I asked myself and God simultaneously. It came in a rush: him drinking with his buddies, having a great time without me doing things that would hurt me—and my mind began to spin out more—him meeting someone when they're out partying while I'm at home being a mom.

The onslaught of fears was real and violent inside me. I was drowning all over again. But then something happened in that moment—an opening, an unclenching of fists, a surrender, or perhaps, grace. I felt myself release my husband. I released him to his own path. I released him to his own choices and his own experiences. I knew whatever choices he would make in his life whether we were together or not, I would be ok, even if it hurt. Surrender, something I had never let go enough to experience—until now on my kitchen floor—poured its deep peace over me.

I think what began to happen for me over time was as I began to release my obsessive grip on his alcoholism, space was created in my life. Space for much needed change. Like opening a window in a stale room and feeling the fresh air envelop me bit by bit, eventually, I was breathing again.

*****

My husband invites me to an open meeting for alcoholics for the first time and I agree to go. I am nervous and curious.

We arrive and as we walk in from the car-lined parking lot, the mellow breeze, cooled off from the daytime warmth, follows us in. The reach of the soft evening light is taking over the sky. It feels expansive tonight, like I can stretch out my arms and take a deep breath and the endless space of the sky itself would fill my lungs and settle in my body.

I've never seen him in a place like this, only heard of him speak of it. Only witnessed the effects of how, over the course of a few years, what they do in this place, slowly turn him inside out and upside down. I've watched the work done here soften and shape him in ways I could have never fathomed. It's become a part of him and it's a land I've never set foot on. But now I'm here, we're here. It feels like more than an arrival at a physical space—the entirety of our beings have arrived here, a winding road trailing behind us.

As we enter the double glass doors, we are greeted with smiles and introductions and handshakes. "Oh, you're Neil's wife! Welcome." I smile genuinely, but also timidly. I'm not sure how to exist here. It's like walking into a room with a crowd of people who all know something you don't.

We approach a table, and I watch his broad shoulders lift the lid off a heavy box full of books. He meticulously places the books on the table for display. I've always appreciated his precise, thorough ways, at times feeling inferior because of them. There are many books with titles like, Welcome Newcomer or For the Family Member of an Alcoholic. He is steady in his movements, calm, happy to be here. He exchanges hugs and jokes with the people around him. I stand at his side and watch him connect from his heart and move with joy. I feel bewildered and intrigued by him, like I did when we first met years ago.

The main room is lit brightly and lined with rows of fold out chairs all facing a speaker stage. His large eyes, whose landscape I've known for nineteen years now, are alive and happy, fringed with long, brown lashes. All these years they've held me in their tumultuous gaze, and I'm remembering that perhaps… I love them.

Different people, men and women, file through the open doors, hugging, laughing, greeting. Their faces, whether young or old, hold eyes full of life and struggle of past and present. Yet somehow, there's something circulating in the air that feels like a secret. A secret you want to know. A secret ablaze, yet steady, grounded. A secret cemented in the depth of human experience one only gains from the wisdom of falling to one's knees.

I've never been to a meeting for alcoholics before. I take my place in one of the chairs, wondering if I really belong here. "It's an open meeting," I'm told. Meaning alcoholics and non-alcoholics alike can attend. The room quiets and people speak, always opening up with, "Hi, I'm Amy and I'm an alcoholic." Or "Hi, I'm George and I'm a Alcoholic." Now, I get to listen to the alcoholic's stories of pain and hope. My husband feels sturdy sitting to my right, his familiar jeans and flannel a comfort to me. It is a nice feeling, a new feeling, sensing his calm strength by my side. Him, who I barred my heart from for years.

It's a curious thing to experience a thawing heart. It came swiftly, seemingly not of my doing, surprising me with its ferocity. It terrified me, this onslaught of emotion towards someone I had felt removed from for years. The pain of our story still rattled its cage around me like a demon.

But something happens when you bring your demons out into the light. It's utterly frightening and heart wrenching and at times, excruciatingly painful. But you get to be free. Even if you lose everything, you get to be free. And I want to be free.

As the meeting comes to a close we say a closing prayer together: God, grant me the serenity to accept the things I cannot change, the courage to change the things I can, and the wisdom to know the difference.

We meander out of the meeting room, out into the star scattered night. People are chatting and laughing on their way to their cars. We make it to ours, and I tilt my head back to take in the night sky, my hair slightly catching the breeze. All the cracks in my armor and the torrent inside me beat life into my imperfect hope, and imperfect faith, and imperfect healing, and I am alive. This work is not done, it never is. And I'm ok with that. We climb into the car, and the headlights illuminate the road before us as we make our way home.

Sometimes I find myself looking around, waiting for something to go wrong. After years of living in a survival state of mind, that leftover, habitual anxiety still catches me. I've found I that I've had to become ok with… being ok. I don't have to scramble around trying to fix the unfixable, or try to hold something together that will never work.

I've found joy and peace in the simplicity of a life where I have nothing to hide, nothing to fight, nothing to force. Learning to care for myself and be accountable for myself keeps me grounded as I tend my side of the street. I am full of awe and gratitude at the capacities of a human being to heal. An unencumbered heart, expansive and open, I've found, is the greatest of gifts.

Thank you for reading my story.

31

ALLISON'S STORY
GUEST AUTHOR

I don't remember my first drink, but I do remember my first drunk. It was my sophomore year of high school and I was visiting my dad for the weekend. I was freshly fourteen and my dad was drinking his fourth martini of the evening when his girlfriend arrived with a four pack of wine coolers. As we sat down to dinner, I asked if I could try one. Everything I'd had before tasted bitter and burned, this tasted like Kool-Aid. By the end of dinner, she had finished one and I had inhaled the other three. With a buzz in me, I asked my dad for another drink, and he provided. From the beginning, I drank to excess. The evening ended with EMT's rushing me to the hospital with a BAC of 0.42.

I was shaken awake the next morning by my mother who quickly ushered in a nurse to remove my IV and handed me a coconut water in its absence. A beverage so simple and refreshing, and yet to this day the taste reminds me of her disappointment. She drove me to school in silence. We didn't talk about anything other than the fact that I might miss first period.

I knew my maternal grandmother had been an alcoholic and that my grandfather went out for a drink one day and never returned. I also knew these were things we didn't talk about. My family did an incredible job of teaching me to look put together on the outside. I made good grades and played varsity sports but none of it brought me joy. The reaction to my juvenile depression was that I needed to eat better, sleep better, be better. I was aware that my parents took it as a personal reflection when I was doing poorly, so I tried to look well. I don't know that I succeeded.

I was pathologically shy in high school. I didn't eat lunch because I couldn't bear eating alone. Instead, I walked laps around campus until the bell rang for us to return to class.

Some time during my senior year, I finally started interacting with my peers. A boy in my English class invited me to a party at the basketball team captain's house. He picked me up and introduced me to a room full of people I had only admired from afar. They offered me a drink and treated me as an equal. My anxiety around others had vanished and I felt happy for the first time since I was a child. I had finally found what made me feel normal; it was alcohol.

For the first time since grade school I had people to eat lunch with, to party with. And that's exactly what I did. Every weekend I drank myself into a blackout, and then somehow, I graduated.

After a summer of daily drinking, I moved to the central coast of California to attend college. I had no interest in excelling in school. Every thought was on meeting people who would supply me with free alcohol. I spent all of my money on substances and Ubers. My first year of college was a blur of blackouts brought on by crippling alcoholism and a pretty severe case of anorexia. By my nineteenth birthday I weighed 70 pounds. I made it halfway through my sophomore year before I developed jaundice, started having chest pains, and passed out walking to class.

As a result I was sent to an eating disorder treatment program. There I started therapy and AA. I spent five months learning self healing and sobriety. When my body appeared well, I stepped down from residential into an intensive outpatient program. Two days after arriving at outpatient, I asked someone to sneak me a bottle of tequila and a ziplock of joints. Three weeks later I was kicked out. I wasn't ready to go back to school, so I went home to disappointed parents. I left every night after dinner and came home just in time for breakfast the next day.

A year later I dragged myself back to campus, still drinking but this time mixing it with a slew of recently prescribed medications that should not be taken with alcohol. After six months I became psychotic and was hospitalized for 17 days. When my mom drove me back to school she told me that if I wanted to stay in contact with my family, I had to go to AA.

I still remember my first meeting. I spent twenty minutes telling my life story to a room full of strangers, and no one interrupted me. Up until this moment most of the people in my life had not been listening to me, just waiting for their turn to speak. Here, absolute strangers were listening to every word I spoke with acceptance.

I developed friendships in AA during my first attempt at sobriety . I became comfortable with my sober life and began to forget what it looked like when I drank. I thought I could moderate, have an occasional beer with a coworker or glass of wine with a friend. We all know how that turned out. I got drunk at a work party and got fired on the spot .

Back to square one. After six more months of hard drinking, I fell into psychosis again. I dropped out of school, lost my apartment, my friends and had already lost my family. I stepped closer to my bottom by deciding to live at the beach. I passed out drunk with a group of strangers and awoke the next morning with my car completely cleaned out of all my possessions including my wallet. I drove to the home of an older man in AA who had taken a liking to me. He had also relapsed, so was happy to provide a warm bed and alcohol to me…in exchange for other services. This quickly devolved into an abusive relationship. During a fight, he knocked me unconscious. I woke up handcuffed in the back of a police car. While they took my mug shot, I realized I had no idea what day it was. I looked at a clock and realized it was my birthday. I turned twenty-two in a jail cell.

The next two years were the definition of insanity. I would gather a few months of sobriety with no step work or sponsor, begin to feel happy, then have the bright idea that a drink would make me even happier. I'd lose myself in a slew of substances and within shorter and shorter durations of time, be involuntarily checked back into the hospital.

For some reason I can only comprehend as God, I still kept coming back. I know a sliver of me wanted to live, wanted sobriety, wanted peace.

A few weeks after my twenty-fourth birthday, I started sharing in meetings that I was in need of a sponsor. I admitted with defeat that I wasn't as smart as I thought I was. I clearly didn't know how to move through life and I needed someone to show me what to do. A young man approached me, and though it wasn't common to be sponsored by the opposite gender, he offered to take on the role until I could find a woman.

He read the book with me and we slowly began to work the steps. It was easy for me to admit I was powerless over alcohol, and even easier to believe that something or someone could restore me to sanity. At this point I had been hospitalized six times and spend the better part of a year of my life in mental facilities because of my drinking and using. I didn't ever want to go back. I was able to speak the sentence that I turned my will over to a higher power but it would take another two years to learn how.

We started my inventory. My life had been the definition of selfish, with a side of chronic victimhood over situations I'd created. My relationships were based upon what I could get from others. For the first time I acknowledged my character defects and made a willing effort to work on them day by day.

Life got better. After seven years of being in and out of school, I was finally able to concentrate long enough to graduate. I got a job that paid decently. I wasn't spending half of my income on alcohol and actually put money into savings. I started taking care of my body and soul. Life got easy and that wasn't something I was used to.

It was difficult at first, getting used to being comfortable. Stress felt like the fuel for my day, and without it, I didn't know what to do.

I started going to the beach, spending hours picking through sand looking for sea glass. This is where I discovered meditation. My mind began to grow quieter and I learned through the universe what it meant to surrender to my surroundings.

When life felt like it was perfect, I lost my job. The thought of taking a drink didn't cross my mind until my now former co-worker handed me a drink and I took it. Like a story straight from the big book, one drink led to another and before I had the sense to stop, I began to vomit. Embarrassed and uncomfortable, I called the man who took me through the steps two years ago, except now he was my partner. He picked me up and took me home. I crawled into bed and cried over losing my time, but I was also deeply grateful. Apparently I needed those final drinks to truly surrender. Without any doubt, I now know that I am an alcoholic. I can not control myself once alcohol enters my body. I can not drink, and I don't want to. I believe that God, the universe, a higher power, or whatever you want to call it handed me that drink. This is a lesson that has been put in front of me time and time again, and even when I thought I'd understood, I hadn't. I needed that lesson to be repeated one final time.

I woke up the next day and went straight to a meeting. I introduced myself as a newcomer and met with my sponsor. We started over at step one. I know without a doubt that I am powerless over alcohol. Today and every day I turn my will over to a higher power. I trust that there is a plan and purpose for me.

I have learned the importance of presence, of being here for myself and the people who have grown to care for me. I have learned there are times I will be wrong, and that all I can do is admit my mistakes and try to learn from them. I am grateful for the lessons I have learned in sobriety, and those shown me during my drinking. Today, when I need help, I ask for it. I realize that relapsing is a part of my story as it is for many recovering alcoholics. Sobriety has brought me clarity, and the ability to enjoy life in the present moment. Now I live just for today, and look at tomorrow as a gift.

THE SOBERING TRUTH

32

ALCOHOLIC AND ADDICTED DOCTORS

His palms were covered with thick scales that were cracked, fissured, and painful, caused by such severe psoriasis that he couldn't use his hands. Roger was one of three principal operators of the Diablo Nuclear Power Plant on the rocky coast near our town. In those hands rested the safety of literally millions.

Miraculously, one of the lesser-known drugs for psoriasis, initially developed to treat malaria and leprosy, cleared up Roger's hands. For twelve years, his hands had been normal and his job secure. Despite that, the psoriasis on the rest of his body worsened. Large, beefy red, scaly plaques covered his forearms and shins. It would just be a while before his hands were unusable again. Perhaps it was time for a change, but the other powerful drugs for psoriasis all had the side effect of liver toxicity.

"Roger, do you drink much?"

"Not at all, Doc."

My medical training and experience of being lied to and disappointed by countless patients left me a little skeptical. I pursued.

"Not at all?"

"No."

"Why not?"

"My dad was an ophthalmologist, and he was a drunk. And when I drank as a young man, I could always see myself becoming like him. So I quit."

"Did you have a problem with it?"

"I could have. I didn't let it go that far."

"Did you go the AA route?"

"No, I just quit."

"What were you like when you drank?"

"I talked too much. It changed me."

"Did it make you mean?"

"No, just different. Alcohol just changes people. They're not the same."

"Your dad was an ophthalmologist?"

"Yeah. And he was drunk every night. He would get argumentative."

"You kept your head down at dinner and left as soon as you finished eating because he wanted to pick a fight?" I had lived through a lot of the same family meals.

"Lots of times, I wouldn't go to dinner. I would lie that I had to study. I would eat in my room and leave him to my brother and my poor mom."

"And she just put up with it?"

"Yeah. What else was she going to do? He was her meal ticket. Besides, lots of people were like that then."

"Still are, but we tolerate it less."

Roger's dad was an HFA. He was a highly successful and respected ophthalmologist. But he drank three double martinis every night, and he died of alcoholic cirrhosis at seventy-three. His children and wife, who had suffered so much punishment over the years, did not mourn much.

Doctors make great drug abusers, especially of alcohol. I don't distinguish between drug abuse and alcoholism because alcohol is a drug. Alcohol is socially accepted, so we don't think of it in the same sense as heroin, speed, or cocaine, but it is no different. My recovering drug abusers from the Liberty Tattoo Program taught me that. A drug is a drug.

Historically, one of the best examples of physicians' vulnerability to drug addiction is William Halstead, a world-famous surgeon, certainly the greatest American doctor of his generation. He was the chief surgeon at Johns Hopkins College of Medicine in Baltimore. He was brilliant, innovative, and dedicated. Many of the surgical procedures and instruments for general surgery still bear his name.

Halstead also discovered the efficacy of cocaine as a local anesthetic. Traveling in South America, he noticed the natives chewing the leaves of the coca plant as they toiled long hours in the hot tropical sun. They seemed to have boundless energy. On occasion, he noticed individuals who accidentally became injured and marveled that they seemed insensitive to the pain of the injury. Halstead began experimenting with an extract of the leaves and found it was a superb local anesthetic, used both topically or injected. As so many physicians did in the early days of modern medicine, he experimented on himself. In the process, he became hopelessly addicted to cocaine. His good friend Henry Firestone, the tire magnate, recognized his problem and arranged a nineteenth-century detox program. He had Halstead kidnapped and put on a steamship headed for Europe. In the two weeks it took to make the voyage, Halstead recovered. He returned to a normal life for several years, but became addicted again later in his life and died an addict.

George Walker was a good ol' boy from Tennessee, a fine surgeon who drank too much. He never drank during the day, but, in the evening, he'd have two or three tall glasses of Tennessee-sipping whiskey. It started innocently enough as social drinking, acceptable at the time, but, as the years passed, his dependence became stronger, the need was greater, and the quantity increased. As happens to so many HFAs, the vortex of the disease trapped George, and he was sucked in.

There were several occasions when he was called in to the emergency room to see patients in the evening, and observant nurses smelled alcohol on his breath. One night, while examining a ten-year-old girl with appendicitis, he was unsteady and slurring his words. Amazingly enough, he operated on her. She recovered uneventfully, but the potential for disaster loomed in the operating room. An unsteady hand could nick the bowel, leading to a fatal peritonitis, or an altered judgment could fail to see a small artery that retracted up into the mesentery, causing the patient to hemorrhage after surgery.

Hospitals and their staffs run like the military. Years ago, nurses would never dare to question a doctor's judgment or physical condition. George's inebriation continued for quite some time until one of the nurses had the courage to say something to another doctor. Once alerted, the doctor made a point of observing George a time or two in the ER after dark. In keeping with the good ol' boy network of doctors, Walker was not reported and referred for therapy. Instead, the chief of surgery mentioned to George at their weekly golf game that alcohol on his breath had been noticed in the ER and he had better be more careful. Also, Walker's partners covered for him, telling the ER staff not to call him in the evening unless they couldn't get in touch with anyone else.

This continued for years. After he retired, his drinking increased and contributed to high blood pressure and a stroke, which killed George in his late sixties. It is amazing how long a person can live with a serious alcohol problem.

Alcoholism still has a social stigma. Our present attitudes toward alcohol are reminiscent of societal views of mental illness a century ago, which espoused that it was a genetic weakness in your family tree never to be revealed. Today, with increased understanding and public education, it is understood that many of these diseases are chemical imbalances or genetic abnormalities to identify and treat. The same must occur with alcoholism. It is a disease, not a character weakness. And once diagnosed, treatment is very effective. Abstention immediately begins to reverse most of the physical and psychiatric damage. Psychotherapy and a twelve-step program usually facilitate insight into the problem, which, along with behavior modification, greatly reduces the chance of relapse.

The medical profession is beginning to see the light. A program now exists in which addicted physicians can enter rehabilitation programs and not lose their licenses. An anonymous hotline is available to report the impaired physician, leading to earlier identification of addicted doctors. The initial motivation may have been fear of liability, but the benefit to patient welfare and safety has become apparent since the advent of the program.

In spite of that, the quarterly bulletin of the California Board of Medical Quality Assurance (BOMQUA) lists twenty to thirty doctors whose licenses have been suspended or revoked due to drug and alcohol abuse. And that's just the tip of the iceberg.

Physicians are bright, and many with addictive problems are very clever and more than a little devious. Take, for instance, Ken Porter, who was a year ahead of me in medical school and close friends with a buddy of mine, Tom Downing. As Tom tells it, the very first day of medical school, this big, handsome guy stuck a huge ham of a hand out at his, and they were fast friends from that day on. He seemed like the nicest guy in the whole world. Later, as Tom began to see Ken's dark side, he was never sure if it had always existed and he had been deceived from the beginning or if the drugs and alcohol had gradually eroded Ken's morality. They studied together, both on Eskatrol. Ken also worked a lot. He was married in his first year, and they had a child by the summer before his second. Attending medical school with a wife and a child on meager funds was tough. Ken needed to work to supplement his grants and loans. When he was a fourth-year student, our hospital was short of interns on obstetrics and gynecology, so they hired fourth-year students to work as interns. Tom worked one night a week. Ken worked two in addition to the time demands of his fourth year. Tom was always amazed at Ken's energy level. As he looks back on it, it was probably pharmacologically induced.

Ken chose internal medicine as a specialty and remained at Los Angeles County. The hours were long, and the work was hard. Ken was incredible. He was never tired and never down. Occasionally, the three of us met socially and drank Rusty Nails, a mixture of scotch and Drambuie, together. Whenever I saw him, I marveled at his stamina and enthusiasm. Everyone I know felt the same about Ken. When something seems too good to be true, it generally is. Ken was probably taking drugs then to maintain the killer pace of his life.

Ken moved with his wife and now-growing family to the central coast a year ahead of me. He actually arranged an interview for me at the clinic where he had taken a job, and his presence in the area was a huge inducement for me to come. After I arrived, we saw less of each other than we had before. I dismissed it as his busy life and a little jealousy on his wife's part. I now realize Ken had parts of his life he didn't want me to see. He worked a killer schedule under the guise of providing for a large and growing family, but loved to spend money.

I started having some doubts about Ken when he mentioned he had his wife on powerful antidepressants. One of the cardinal rules in medicine is that physicians, ethically speaking, should not treat themselves or their families, as it clouds their judgment, and it is taboo. Why would Ken choose to diagnose and treat his wife? Why was she depressed?

Then Ken left his clinic under a cloud of controversy. His contract provided that all his income would be shared with the group, yet he had been doing a lot of outside consulting and keeping the money. Ken believed he was practically supporting the clinic with his office income and they had no right to any more. The clinic stated that Ken breached his contract.

Being the good friend, I helped Ken move his desk and files out of the clinic on a weekend before they had a chance to lock him out. He was my friend, and I supported him. I did not suspect that his drug use might be eroding his ethical judgment.

After Ken left the clinic, he opened his own office, and his practice flourished. To this day, ten years later, patients we had in common will tell you that he was the best doctor they ever had. And he was. But he left his wife for a nurse he met at the hospital, and many rumors circulated it was not the first or even the tenth.

He deserted his staff with a startling suddenness. Employees of two decades were left without a job or any retirement provision. One of his nurses came in to see me a while back, and she was still in shock at the way she had been treated. Without rancor, she recounted how she gradually discovered that Ken had a drug abuse problem. She finally confronted him with it and threatened to turn him in. He was more careful about not letting her see his problem until he finally left town.

I asked how he managed to do it. She said he was masterful at regulating his level of consciousness. When he was tired, he took uppers. When he was wired, he took downers. He had the right drug for the right mood.

Can people do that for a lifetime? Maybe he'll get away with it. Or perhaps he'll end up like Eric Cavanaugh, a brilliant man, one of the smartest men I ever met. He was multitalented, a fine athlete with a keen mind and shrewd business savvy. Like Roger Tate's dad, Eric was an ophthalmologist. He trained at the best schools. By all accounts, he had excellent clinical judgment when it came to patients.

But he had a drinking and a drug problem. Eric was one of those people to whom everything came too easily. He was the kind of student who never had to study and aced the tests anyway. Eric would quickly master a subject or sport and then become bored. He was always looking for the next challenge, the next adrenaline rush. In research science or some field of inquiry with unlimited questions and the right direction, Eric could have been a great scientist or a Nobel Prize winner. But his prime motivation was money and status, and he had a fatal flaw. He believed he could drink and experiment with drugs and not get burned.

There's no telling when the serious problems began. When I met him, he was sixty, and he had clearly been compromised for at least a decade. He drank hard every evening. His adult children refused to have dinner with him or stop by in the evening because he got drunk and ugly. But he also self-medicated with uppers and downers and whatever was the latest psychoactive drug on the market. He mixed and matched. The arrogant are particularly subject to the seduction of drugs and alcohol because they think they are too smart to get into trouble. They'll recognize a problem developing, and they are strong enough to overcome the addiction. It's not going to happen to them.

Almost imperceptibly, Eric began to slip with a bill unpaid here, a critical clause in a contract not read there, and a flawed business decision made now that never would have occurred ten years before. And there were moments of confusion. Eric would awaken at night, confused at his surroundings. He was subject to dreadful nightmares. Within five years, Eric gradually spiraled into profound dementia. As of this writing, he is in a locked facility and doesn't recognize his wife or children. He has coarse tremors and a wide-based, staggering gate, and he is deteriorating rapidly. There is no other family history of dementia.

What happens to brain cells when they are so radically altered by alcohol and psychoactive drugs? Critical brain chemicals, the neurotransmitters, are produced in greater or lesser amounts and become depleted in some areas of the brain. The normal release and reuptake is changed forever. This system is very complex and in delicate balance, and our emotional and mental health is completely dependent on it. Drinking and doing drugs negatively alter this necessary balance.

THE SOBERING TRUTH

33

OBSERVATIONS OF A HIGHWAY PATROL OFFICER

Officer Chuck Margaroli has worked for the California Highway Patrol for thirty years. He has arrested countless drunk drivers and seen innumerable auto accidents with injuries and fatalities caused by intoxicated drivers.

I asked him candidly what he'd like to see change about our drunk-driving laws or the way they are enforced. He responded that the decreased tolerance for the drunk driver, both by the public and law enforcement, is a positive change that's long overdue. Yet, those who are outraged by a driver with a blood alcohol level of 0.24 percent who drives the wrong direction on the freeway and kills a mother and her two young children in a head-on collision will drive home from a party with a blood alcohol level of 0.12 percent without a second thought. It's always someone else who has the drinking problem. Chuck would like to see people wake up that it's their problem, too.

Chuck has noticed a significant increase in drunk driving since the terrorist attacks of September 11. He attributes it to general anxiety in the community about the future safety of our country and our world.

The law enforcement community's focus on holiday drinking has decreased drunk driving on the holidays themselves, through a heightened public awareness of consequences and increased use of designated drivers. But it's not just Thanksgiving, Christmas, and New Year's Eve that are the problem. It's the entire holiday season. Drunken driving arrests and accidents increase throughout, beginning at Thanksgiving and continuing through New Year's Day. He attributes holiday parties for fueling the problem.

Officer Margaroli is pleased with the stringent laws punishing drunk drivers, notably the enhanced penalties for driving under the influence with a child (under fourteen) in the vehicle, the enhanced penalties for having a blood alcohol level in excess of 0.20 percent, and the mandatory jail term for a fourth offense. But he is frustrated with the judicial system's enforcement of the laws, particularly judges who throw out solid cases on legal technicalities. They have cast doubt repeatedly on his or other officers' judgment, and they have implied the officer was overzealous in his pursuit of a particular case or he may have bent the truth in order to establish certain evidence. For example, on one occasion, Officer Margaroli and his partner were parked at a stop sign on the outskirts of one of the South County beach cities. A lady returning home after an afternoon of golf and evening of drinking at the nearby country club literally skidded through the stop sign and intersection in front of them. They stopped her for running the stop sign. They observed somewhat intoxicated behavior while interviewing her. She failed field sobriety tests and blew a 0.18 percent blood alcohol level on the preliminary alcohol screening (PAS) device. Chuck and his partner arrested her. At the jail, she blew a 0.16 percent blood alcohol level on the more accurate and court-admissible intoxicimeter.

This case of intoxication while driving was dismissed. The defendant's attorney submitted a weather report stating there was dense fog that night. He insisted the officers could not possibly have observed the defendant skidding through the stop sign, that they did not have probable cause to stop her. He filed a motion to suppress all the evidence of her intoxication that was gleaned subsequent to her being stopped. Officer Margaroli explained the fog was patchy and they had a clear view of the intersection, but the judge threw out the case on the attorney's motion. That needs to stop.

Officer Margaroli also would like to see a relatively new defense strategy called the rising blood alcohol defense disallowed. Say, for instance, a driver is stopped, is judged to show signs of intoxication, and blows a 0.08 percent blood alcohol level. At the jail, he blows a 0.10 percent blood alcohol level, and he is booked for drunk driving. The attorneys will argue the defendant had a drink just before the arrest and the alcohol was still being assimilated. Because it was barely the legal limit for intoxication at the time it was checked, it was actually lower than when the defendant was stopped, so the defendant was not legally intoxicated.

Our veteran patrolman vigorously applauds the zero-tolerance policy for minors. Under the present laws, anyone under twenty-one may have no alcohol in his blood. If he does, it is an automatic two-year suspension of his driver's license. Because teen drinking is a persistent and growing problem, it doesn't keep young people from drinking, but it has gone a long way toward keeping them off the road when they have been drinking.

When I asked him to cite the drunk-driving case that he remembered most vividly, he recounted a story of a local dentist who had been drinking at a seaside bar. Driving home at a high rate of speed, he lost control of his vehicle on a tight turn called "screech owl curve," well known for the many accidents that have occurred there. His car crossed the center divider and hit an oncoming compact car. The dentist was driving a large Mercedes. Although it was nearly totaled, he was unhurt. Miraculously, the driver of the compact was not killed, but he sustained massive injuries including two broken legs, a dislocated shoulder, and extensive facial fractures and lacerations.

The dentist had a blood alcohol level in excess of 0.20 percent. He pleaded no contest to driving under the influence. By doing this, he is not admitting guilt in a civil suit that could follow the criminal action of his drunk-driving trial. The victim spent years enduring reconstructive surgery and rehabilitating his extensive orthopedic injuries. He will never return to his pre-accident state and will carry the scars and pains of his injuries for the remainder of his life. The dentist, virtually unscathed, was sentenced to a six-month license suspension and attendance at alcohol school, in addition to his automobile insurance premiums rising $2,000 a year. What's wrong with this picture?

Recently, a drunk driver killed a police dispatcher from our local university. The dispatcher was stopped at a signal on Highway One when a drunk driver, oblivious to the stopped vehicle, slammed into the back of her car. The force of the impact severed the spine of the stationary driver, and she died of her massive injuries after a week in the intensive care unit of a local hospital. The drunk driver had a blood alcohol level of 0.17 percent, and this was his sixth offense for drunk driving.

When I asked the patrolman how a five-time offender was allowed back on the road, he simply answered, "We don't allow him. He was driving on a revoked license."

The driver, tried for vehicular manslaughter, was convicted. The original sentence was seven years, which was later increased to eleven on the special circumstances of repeat offenses. How can we get these repeat offenders off the road? If they disregard the law and drive drunk on suspended and revoked licenses, perhaps they need to be incarcerated to protect the population against their public menace.

After thirty years on the job, Officer Margaroli knows when to expect several drunks on the road. Sunny weekends are always bad. The beer starts flowing after noon. By mid-to-late afternoon, when the cowboys are all heading home, most of them have a snoot full. Given that a lot of drinking starts in the mid-to-late afternoon and continues into the evening, the peak times for drunk drivers is five o'clock to eleven o'clock on the weekends. Another significant time period is just after two o'clock in the morning when the bars close.

Asked which drunk drivers are the most difficult to handle, the officer is automatic in his response. "It's the women. They are all sweetness and light when first stopped, certain they can flirt their way out of an arrest. When it is apparent that arrest is inevitable, they turn into witches or worse."

Officer Margaroli reports that the vilest language he has ever heard came from the mouth of the same woman who, five minutes before, was the picture of decorum.

Asked what was the highest blood alcohol he has ever seen in his long career, he relates a story of an arrest he made within the last decade. He was making a traffic stop for a speeding driver. Pulled to the side of the road with the previously speeding vehicle, the officer noticed a car pull up behind him. A man got out and staggered toward him. Slurring his words, the man asked for directions to a location several miles down the road. After a brief interview and failed field sobriety tests, the man blew into the PAS apparatus. The patrolman was astounded to see the results, 0.36 percent. Most with a blood alcohol level at that level would be barely conscious, certainly not upright and walking. Chuck arrested the man and took him to jail, but he could not be prosecuted for drunk driving because he was not observed driving, only drunk in public, a much less serious offense.

Officer Margaroli has some sage advice for anyone who would drink and drive. "Don't do it. You may escape notice for years, but the slightest error may send a ton-and-a-half of steel careening off the highway or into another vehicle. You may be charged with murder or at least vehicular manslaughter. Imagine living with the guilt of injuring or killing someone. Have someone else, someone sober, drive you home before you see those flashing red lights in your rearview mirror and your life changes forever."

THE SOBERING TRUTH

34

SCOTT

My friend Scott died last night. A self-destructive force he set in motion twenty-five years ago, a squamous cell cancer, finally had its way.

He grew up a good kid and talented athlete in Santa Cruz, California. Never a gifted student, he drifted toward manual skills in high school--wood shop, metal shop, and auto shop. There was no hint of the tragedy to come.

Unfortunately, he chose the wrong friends in high school. They drank beer, and he joined in. He stopped attending church and drifted away from his family and their values. Scott progressed from beer to cocaine. As so often happens, the alcohol and drugs consumed him. He borrowed money from drug dealers, who take a dim view of addicts who skip out on their debts. He stole from his parents, abandoning his sense of right to the demands of his addiction. Finally, with a warrant out for his arrest and some unsavory characters looking for him, Scott cowered in a flophouse closet, contemplating suicide. In desperation, he called home instead. His dad would speak with him only at their pastor's house. When he arrived, the ultimatum given was detox or jail.

Scott spent a month in an inpatient recovery center in Monterey. That's where, on his first day, he met our mutual friend, Bud. Just out of DTs, Bud was trying to negotiate his way down the hall, but, still heavily medicated, he needed the wall for balance. Scott saw this disheveled person sliding along a wall coming toward him, never dreaming they'd become lifelong friends. They roomed together, and they were soul and accountability friends ever since. As Bud likes to put it, Scott was "present at the creation."

Scott was one of the lucky ones, an addict who didn't die. Of the thirty people at the recovery center with Bud and Scott, only five are still alive. The rest succumbed to their recurrent addictions or committed suicide, attributable to the hopelessness of their failed attempts to remain clean and sober. Scott succeeded in his recovery and built a wonderful life. He married Peggy, channeled his obsessive nature into a passion for fishing, and worked as a building contractor known for his honesty and excellent product. He accomplished this through a reborn faith and continued participation in a twelve-step program.

The goal of recovery is not sobriety. It is contentment. Many recovering alcoholics are sober, but they don't progress past abstinence to the attainment of peace. These dry drunks haven't faced and solved the many personal issues that fueled their addiction. They are simply abstinent. Scott progressed beyond sober to content. He was a genuinely happy person, and he had a wonderful sense of humor with clever perceptions that only enlighten a soul who has traveled to perdition and back. I am so privileged to have known Scott and to have shared his insights into drug and alcohol abuse. It's ironic that I was acquainted with Scott for several years before his illness, but didn't really get to know him until he got sick. Coincidentally, that was just before I gave up drinking. Until I was sober, his resolve intimidated me. Only someone with the problem can appreciate the strength of someone in recovery. Once I was sober, I felt perfectly comfortable being with and getting to know Scott. It was a remarkable experience.

Unfortunately, ten years of heavy drinking and smoking took a toll. Once a person sets in motion a destructive force, and it progresses beyond a certain point, say to the development of a virulent cancer, it cannot be recalled. So it was with Scott. Three years ago, he came in for a checkup and showed me a lump on the right side of his neck, which he had noticed a week before. It was firm but not rock-hard, and I thought it might simply be an enlarged lymph node from a prior sore throat. When it didn't diminish in two weeks on antibiotics, I referred him to an ear, nose, and throat specialist for a needle biopsy. It was inconclusive, but suspicious for malignancy. What followed was an excisional biopsy, where the entire lump was removed and immediately examined with frozen sections. It turned out to be squamous cell cancer, metastatic to a lymph node in Scott's neck. As a result, at the time of the biopsy, Scott had a radical neck dissection, a ghastly procedure where all the lymph nodes and major muscles of the left side of his neck were removed. At the same time, his mouth, throat, larynx, upper bronchi, and esophagus were examined with an endoscope. In an attempt to find the primary cancer site, fifteen small biopsies were taken from unusual-looking areas. The final results showed cancer in three of the neck nodes, but no definitely positive site that could be called the primary site. As you have already learned, the combination of heavy drinking and smoking are prime causes of squamous cancer of all the areas suspected of harboring Scott's primary.

Following the surgery, Scott had intense radiation to his neck and upper chest for six weeks, causing his throat to become so sore that he couldn't eat. A feeding tube was placed through his upper abdomen into his stomach, which remained for three months after the treatments ended. He lost thirty pounds and never recovered his sense of taste or salivary gland function. He lived with a bottle of water in one hand and sipped on it constantly to moisten his radiation-burned mouth and throat.

There was a six-month period of relatively good health. Scott got back to work, and his days off and weekends reaped a rich harvest of salmon, halibut, and sea bass. He was happy. With each passing day, it looked as if he might beat this deadly foe. Then a routine scan showed a spot in his lung and several in his liver. The lung they could radiate, but not the liver, so Scott began an additional five weeks of radiation and intravenous infusions of chemotherapy, which left him very weak and nauseous. He lost another twenty pounds. Through it all, he worked and fished.

Last summer, I was planning my first fishing trip to Alaska, accompanied by my best friend and son-in-law. At the last minute, I thought of including Scott. I checked with our host in Alaska. Assured it was no problem to include another fisherman, I asked Scott.

"Have you ever been to Alaska, Scott?"

"No, but I have always wanted to go."

"I'm going in a month with Hurley and Steven. Want to go?"

I will never forget the light in Scott's eyes as he considered the fulfillment of a lifelong dream.

"I'd love to," he said simply. And it was done.

Several weeks before we left, Scott began to develop severe headaches. Almost paralyzing and migraine-like, they made even the simplest of tasks nearly impossible. They were explained as a side effect of his chemotherapy. A combination of powerful pain medication and a relatively new migraine medicine made them almost tolerable, but a single dose of the migraine medication was $30, and Scott had no health insurance.

Alaska was beautiful beyond words. Blue-green mirrorlike passages were dotted with fir-covered islands. Whales breached beside the boat. Bald eagles warily watched from the bleached tops of lifeless pines. Scott, the consummate fisherman, was in his element. He and our host, Dave, compared notes on everything from reels to filleting knives. And the first one to land a fish, a beautiful halibut, was Scott. Despite a little nausea, a delayed side effect of the chemo, Scott had a beautiful twenty-five-pound king salmon, a limit of three halibut, and several snapper within two hours of reaching the fishing grounds. I remember so well the look of happiness and contentment on his face as we motored in through the glassy inland waterways, headed home. Each of the three days we fished was magical for Scott, but he fought mightily against the pounding in his head. And when he had the headaches, he could hardly function. With effort, we arrived home with a beaming Scott and a hundred pounds of frozen halibut and salmon.

The day after we returned, an MRI of Scott's brain confirmed my suspicions. It showed two tumors: one golf ball-sized behind his right eye (the site of the headaches) and the other marble-sized in the brain stem at the base of the brain. The first was operable. The second was not, but it could be treated with radiation. That same night, the frontal tumor was removed. Five days after the surgery, Scott began radiation. Miraculously, the headaches disappeared. Scott was soon hairless on his scalp, but the radiation oncologist guaranteed Scott he could save his beard. A form-fitting lead shield was constructed to maintain his facial hair. I shaved my head a bit closer than usual in solidarity with Scott. Instead of having bad hair days, we laughed that we had "no hair days."

The radiation and chemo destroyed the brain tumors, but there was ever-growing concern about the tumors in the liver and around the kidneys. Scott would undergo chemo once a week, a four-hour intravenous infusion of poisons designed to kill the rapidly growing cells of the tumor in preference over the normal cells of his body. Unfortunately, the poisons can't tell the bad cells from the good. Any rapidly growing cells, such as bone marrow, skin, hair, and cells lining the gastrointestinal tract, are susceptible to the chemotherapy. For two days after the chemo, Scott would feel reasonably okay. Then he'd become very ill. The principal side effect was an intractable nausea.

"Like the worst seasick you've ever imagined," Scott would explain.

Ironically, he'd never been seasick a day in his life. He took pride in the fact that he could fish the roughest seas and never have a problem. But the chemo was different. There were drugs to ease the nausea, but they had their own set of side effects. Some caused extreme drowsiness; some caused involuntary twitching and contraction of muscles. Still others caused headaches.

Through it all, Scott kept working, fishing, and going to AA meetings. He had a number of jobs in progress. He was too weak to work a full day at his normal pace, so several good friends in the building business pitched in and helped him complete them. He bought a fancy new used boat with a friend. Together, they revamped it and took it on some weekend excursions to the Sacramento River Delta for striped bass and sturgeon.

But Scott was losing his battle against cancer. The repeated scans showed more numerous and larger tumors, and the nausea and weakness were exhausting. Scott quit chemo and tried an alternative herbal treatment, but the herbs made him as sick as the chemo. Fighter that he was, he never stopped looking for an answer. Having beat alcohol and cocaine addiction sixteen years before, he felt he could beat anything.

He had just started yet another chemo when he turned yellow and the pain started in earnest. The liver tumors were obstructing bile ducts, backing the bile up into the circulation and making him jaundiced. And the blockage of the ducts caused pain similar to an attack of gallstones.

Physicians know biliary colic to be one of the most excruciating pains that patients experience.

With each crescendo of pain, Scott's oncologist responded with a stronger and more effective medication. But the liver blockage also increased the ammonia and other toxins in Scott's blood, causing him to gradually lose his grip on reality. Ironically, although Scott's sixteen years of sobriety meant he would never die of liver failure from alcohol, he was to die from liver failure caused by his squamous cancer.

With each passing day, Scott became more yellow, gaunter, and a bit more infantile. In bed, he made strange grimacing expressions. Lying on his back, he picked at his bedclothes as if they had small specks of lint on them. He disassembled the fax machine trying to fix what wasn't broken. His wife or one of the family members had to watch him constantly as he roamed the house because he would fix the computer, the television, his fishing gear, and the coffeemaker.

He stopped eating and drank only small sips when prompted or when medication was required. After what seemed an eternity, he finally went to bed for the last time while his strong, young heart and body fought death for three long days.

Cancer won the corporal battle. Scott won the spiritual battle, however, and the battle over his addiction. When our dear mutual friend, Bud, spoke at his memorial, he announced Scott had attained a lifetime goal they each had from the beginning, from the creation of their sobriety. He had died sober.

And Scott would not have us mourn his passing. He had lived sixteen years beyond the closet, saved by the love and support of skilled and insightful people. Scott had created a rich, new life working, fishing, loving, and sharing his story with anyone who would listen. It's just that his second life was too short. Scott died two months and twenty-three days short of his forty-fifth birthday.

35

I HAVE AN EXCUSE

He sat trembling, pulling little scabs off the back of his hand. He'd hold them up to me as proof of the worms he had seen crawling out of his skin.

"See. Here's one of them. Now you'll believe me."

Ronnie had delusions of parasitosis, believing he had critters burrowing out of his skin. It is a disease characteristically caused by specific drug abuse.

"Is it coke or meth, Ronnie?"

"It's crank, doc. And booze."

"Aren't you tired of being a slave to it? It owns you."

"Yeah, doc, I am. Maybe sometime I'll quit, but not right now. There's too much stress. I can't get over losing my dad."

"There's always gonna be something, Ronnie."

"Doc, you'd drink and do crank, too, if you'd been through what I've been through."

One of the common story threads of the majority of alcoholics is that they drink for good reason and it is almost never their fault. In medical school and throughout my medical career, I've noticed alcoholics as a group can always justify their behavior. With apologies to my psychologist/psychiatrist colleagues, I divide much of the world's psychopathology into two personality types: neurosis and character disorder.

- Neurotics blame themselves for everything. If Grandma fell and broke her hip at the nursing home, it was because the neurotic person forgot to call her that day.

- People with a character disorder are just the opposite. It's never their fault. If they run a red light and broadside someone in an intersection, it's because the sun blinded them through the windshield and they couldn't see the signal. So they sue the city for placing the signal improperly. Alcohol abusers fit in the latter category, as a rule. Their drinking and behavior it produces is not their fault.

Harold was a career alcoholic. I admitted him twice during my stint on the overdose ward at LA County-USC Medical Center. As he sobered up, he always would get weepy and blubber about how it was all her fault. He was referring to his wife, Sarah, who left him after five years of marriage because she couldn't live with his drinking. He'd been through three jobs, had been in the detox unit five times, and had two DUIs. Sarah went through counseling, joined Al-Anon, and got Harold into an alcohol rehab program, but eventually felt Harold didn't want to quit, so she opted out of their marriage. It is a startling revelation for the loved one to discover the alcoholic chooses alcohol over his mate. But given the nature of addiction, it is true. The sooner the alcoholic's spouse comes to that realization and separates herself, the better. By staying with the alcoholic and praying he will recover, she is enabling him to continue drinking. By leaving him, she is appropriately attaching negative consequences to the addiction. Sarah prayed the initial separation and possible conditional return would be the motivation

Harold needed to quit. It was not. It simply provided him with a reason to continue drinking. Whatever previous excuse Harold used before his separation, forever after, it was the cruelty of his wife leaving him that created his grief. And it really was unquenchable, first with vodka and whiskey. Later, when he really hit the skids, it was with cheap port and Tokay. The divorce made drinking so much easier for Harold, as he rationalized that it was his wife's fault. His grief was so overwhelming that it was uncontrollable. He had to drink. Notice how subtly Harold had changed the argument. His drinking was not the problem. It was the grief, and Sarah was to blame.

Joe was an alcoholic I treated during my residency at the VA hospital

I HAVE AN EXCUSE

in Long Beach. He had terrible psoriasis. Half of his body was covered with huge, red, scaly patches. For the uninitiated, the appearance of severe psoriasis is grotesque. These patients have a terrible social stigma, and many of them drink to try to cope with their feelings of denigration. As I explained previously, ironically, heavy drinking exacerbates psoriasis. So the binges and flares of psoriasis go hand in hand. In fact, scientific papers have looked at whether alcoholism might trigger the onset or flaring of psoriasis in susceptible individuals.

Joe would come in after two weeks of hard drinking. His psoriasis would be out of control and oftentimes secondarily infected with strep or staph bacteria. I would dry him out, treat the infection, put him in our ultraviolet light cabinet, get his psoriasis well on the way to clearing up, and then send him out to repeat the cycle all over again.

"You don't know what it's like, doc. My life is hell. You should try to live with this crap."

And he was right. I didn't know. Thirty years later, I have taken care of hundreds of patients with psoriasis, and I know it is one of life's great challenges. But I take care of some very high-profile state and local officials, a very successful attorney, several physicians, and many other highly successful people with psoriasis who don't need to use it as an excuse to drink. They meet the challenge. In conquering it, they make the other challenges in their lives more attainable.

Alcoholics will use any excuse as a justification for their problem. One of the worst drunks I treated at LA County-USC was a woman in her mid-thirties whose life spun out of control after she lost a baby to a third-trimester miscarriage in her mid-twenties. She drank heavily during the pregnancy, and her grief at the loss may have been mixed with a large dose of subconscious guilt at perhaps contributing to the stillbirth. It may have been a blessing that she did lose the baby. If she had carried it to term, the child quite possibly would have had fetal alcohol syndrome.

There are untold numbers of alcoholics who were unloved or abused as children or who are drunk because they hate work or lost their job. Perhaps they flunked out of medical school, lost the big promotion, or a close family member died of cancer. Any negative circumstance is an excuse to drink. They so brilliantly change the focus from their drinking to some life-altering event that caused them to drink. Then they are not to blame.

Most alcohol abusers believe that drinking helps them to cope with their difficult lives. Alcohol doesn't help anyone cope with anything. At the end of the first or second drink, there is a feel-good moment that produces a nanosecond of bliss, but it is followed by stupor and, in time, depression. If you add depression to whatever it is that originally created the need to drink, the problem only gets worse.

36

REACTIVE DRINKING

He bent to the task and pulled the skiff in on the long rope. His movements were quick, and his strength was astonishing. The bottom scraped on the rocky shore as the boat grounded. At seventy-four, Rick moved like a man half his age. He had been a lumberjack and roustabout in Alaska for thirty years and an alcoholic for fifty. Five decades of drinking and fighting left little of Jack's dentition.

A buddy of mine hired him to help build a dock. The night before, Rick had beached his boat at three o'clock in the morning, staggered out, fell on the rocks, and then crawled home. Amazingly, he was there at seven o'clock to start work, showing no apparent sign of the previous night's debauch. How can he drink that hard and still function the next day?

There are several good explanations. The first and most logical is that he doesn't function nearly as well as he would if he had not been plastered the night before. Rick's liver could not have metabolized all the alcohol he'd consumed the previous night by the time he arrived at work. He still has a significant blood alcohol level at seven o'clock. So how does he function? Simply put, Rick functions at a reasonably effective level still drunk, with a blood alcohol level of 0.1 to 0.2 percent. It is a learned skill, like driving drunk. Many people can drive well enough not to be spotted by the highway patrol with a blood alcohol level in that range. On tests of subtle motor skills or reaction times, results are abnormal. Nevertheless, many function well enough to get by. And, of course, as the blood alcohol level drops and symptoms of withdrawal arise, Rick starts drinking again.

The amazing fact, for many people like Rick, is that they are virtually never sober ... ever.

How can he maintain a high level of alcohol intake for fifty years and not have cirrhosis? There are many reasons. It may depend on what he drinks. Beer is relatively liver-friendly because it doesn't contain a lot of impurities. Distilled spirits are a lot more toxic to the liver. Distillation is the process of boiling a liquid that has been fermented to produce alcohol. The alcohol has a lower boiling point, so it boils before water and is concentrated. However, in the distillation process, many other volatile chemicals such as benzene and toluene are concentrated as well. Many are more toxic to the liver than alcohol is. As a result, drinking distilled spirits may render the drunk more likely to develop cirrhosis.

Jack avoided or postponed liver disease by eating well when he drank. Liver cells have an amazing ability to regenerate, but they require a significant amount of protein and vitamins in the diet. If absent, the same amount of alcohol causes more damage because the liver doesn't repair itself as well. Alcoholics may not eat much because they are too drunk to care, or the alcoholic calories satisfy their hunger. When alcohol intake creates a nutritional deficiency, the process of cirrhosis is accelerated.

Finally, there appears to be genetic susceptibility to cirrhosis. Two people can drink the same type and amount of alcohol and have the same diet. One develops cirrhosis; the other doesn't. One liver simply doesn't repair as well as the other after injury from alcohol. Or perhaps more scar tissue is made. It's similar to emphysema and smoking. Some people develop the devastating lung disease with light smoking while others, like my uncle, can smoke two packs a day for sixty years and not even be short of breath.

The situation with alcohol is not understood as well, but it must have a similar mechanism. Some people repair their alcoholic hepatitis more efficiently, with less scar tissue, than others. Rick, the lumberjack, obviously does. It appears Rick has a genetically acquired resistance to alcoholic liver disease.

But there's a lot more to Rick than a toothless, drunk lumberman. He has a remarkable intellect. Sometime between work and nightly intoxication, Rick reads voraciously. He checked out books at the library and devoured them. He could discuss any of the great classics in depth. Considering he was drunk most of the time, how did he read, digest, and remember all those books? Rick may represent the 1 percent of the population who can drink excessively and function both physically and intellectually at a very high level. Again, it may be attributed to incredible genes. Yet what a loss to society! Rick could have been an inspiring teacher or writer. To see an intellect such as his wasted on drunken discussions of Hamlet is a shame.

Curiosity about Rick's life choices is heightened by the knowledge that he has two brothers, both of whom are very accomplished. One is a prominent physician in the Boston area; the other is a CEO of a NASDAQ company. Clearly, Rick didn't get all the brains, but he got his share. Why did he choose to squander this gift? Rick was the youngest of three brothers. It is a common scenario in the dynamics of family life that second and third siblings, feeling they cannot successfully compete with an older and very accomplished sibling, choose alternate goals, lifestyles, and pathways. That is certainly the case with Rick. Under the guise of his alcoholism, he simply refused to compete with his older brothers.

Alcohol often serves a psychological need in the beginning. Once the addiction is well established, it maintains a life of its own. Many alcoholics drink to ease psychic pain resulting from lack of parental love, lack of self-esteem, death of a loved one, or a broken marriage. The long list of precipitating factors can also include estranged parents or children, physical pain and disability, shyness, disappointment at not fulfilling a life goal, or, for the overly empathetic, the inability to cope with the great pain and sorrow in our society. The world has always been replete with pain and suffering. There has always been injustice, poverty, illness, hatred, and evil. It is not a question of whether we will experience pain or not, but how we deal with it.

In America, we live in a fix-it culture. It is often thought that our modern technological world has the solution to any problem. If we can reprogram a satellite a hundred miles into space, we should be able to solve our problems here on earth. We expect solutions. Being the impatient people we are, we want the solution right now. We are also a feel-good society. Great social significance is placed on being happy, being fulfilled, and finding meaning in life. So, in summary, we want and expect happiness right now. We want to understand why we are not happy, and we want and expect to fix it right now.

And when these expectations are not met, what do we do? We change jobs. We get a divorce. We get angry. We drink or take drugs. We escape from the problem. We are not willing to endure the stress, pain, or conflict and let it temper us. We are not willing to accept that there is no immediate answer and we simply have to be with the problem a while to let it transform us into stronger, humbler, and more serene people. We are not willing to be humbled by the problem. We are not willing to ask for help outside of ourselves. So we have higher-than-ever rates of divorce, suicide, alcoholism and drug abuse, violent crime, spousal and child abuse, dissatisfaction, and medical illness.

Sadly, alcohol never solves the problem. It just eases the pain for a time. When we sober up, it remains unsolved. As an AA friend put it, "Your life can never be so messed up that alcohol can't make it worse."

NEVER SOBER

If you drink every day, you are never completely sober, completely without the effect of alcohol in your system. There are spaces within the body where fluids exist, the constituents of which are altered very slowly. The aqueous humor in the front or anterior chamber of the eye and the vitreous humor behind the lens are two such spaces. Alcohol is removed very slowly from these areas, so slowly in fact that forensic pathologists can measure the alcohol level in these fluids postmortem and determine, with great accuracy, the blood alcohol level and state of sobriety or inebriation of the deceased for several days before death. Alcohol also persists in isolated areas of the brain and in alterations to the chemical messengers in nerve cells. So, for many who drink every day, they are always under the influence.

37

BUD

He looked and acted the part. He was tan and athletic with a keen mind and a friendly handshake. A triathlete who also completed double-century bike races, he was a noted professor of history at our local university. And no matter what time of the day, he always smelled of liquor. I marveled at how he could do it, and I noted he was increasingly inebriated each time I saw him in the office. Then he suddenly disappeared. He had serious skin cancer problems, and I saw him regularly every three months. When his appointments stopped, I figured he must have changed doctors or maybe died of alcoholism. Almost.

When Bud Beecher returned for a visit, the tan had faded, and he had lost some weight. He had the look of a man who had been to the edge, looked over, and decided not to jump. He was sober.

Bud had come perilously close to killing himself with alcohol, but, in the critical moment approaching self-destruction, his psychologist orchestrated an intervention. Bud entered a recovery and rehabilitation program and joined AA, and he was rescued from alcoholic meltdown.

That was twenty-three years ago. Since then, he has completed a master's in psychology and become a successful drug and alcohol counselor. Retired from teaching history and mentoring aspiring teachers, he has dedicated his life to helping alcoholics understand their addiction and learn to find contentment in an increasingly psychotic world. He wants to help save them from certain destruction. He mentored me. Previously unaware of my drinking problem, he heard a lot about my past life once I quit for good. With the unique perspective of a recovering alcoholic psychologist, Bud had many answers to help me understand the dynamics of my alcoholism.

Bud was born into a lower middle-class, blue-collar family in the early 1940s. His dad was a mechanic; his mother was a stay-at-home mom. Neither was highly educated or emotionally mature. His was a no-talk family. Bud described it as one of those households with an elephant in the living room. A casual observer would take one look at the family interaction and say, "What are you doing with that elephant in the living room?" Everybody in the family would say, "What elephant?" Denial and inability to express emotions characterized this quiet, depressed, and angry household.

In the second grade, Bud went on a class field trip to his first play, *The Emperor's New Clothes*. It was an epiphany. He saw the beauty of the costumes, complexity of the story, and pageantry of a stage production, and he was captivated. A door had been opened on his dark, narrow existence, and Bud immediately fell in love with performance art.

The experience motivated him to read classics such as Dante's *Inferno* and *A Streetcar Named Desire*. He emptied the shelves of the local library, but his extracurricular reading didn't make him a good student. At his high school, there was no incentive to achieve, and teachers didn't care as long as their students weren't fighting. For Bud, there was no life outside of Norwalk. Working after school as an apprentice mechanic despite a burgeoning intellect, Bud prepared for a life in his father's image.

In February 1958, Bud had another awakening. He didn't want to follow his fellow students to prison or make any life-altering mistakes. He had been dating a sleazy girl with sexual experience. One night, they borrowed a car and some liquor and got really drunk. Bud woke up the next morning to the realization he may have ruined his life. He recognized that alcohol made him do things he didn't want to do, and he swore it off. He dropped the girl and his hoodlum friends and searched for a way out of his lifestyle.

He found her on a sunny beach one Sunday. Her name was Nellie, and she came from an impoverished and rigid Lutheran background. Nellie's father was disabled and unable to care for his family. His children were farmed out to relatives. Nellie, at fifteen, was working as a live-in maid for a cousin. She wasn't supposed to be on the beach that Sunday, as recreation on the Sabbath was a sin. But she was. And so was Bud. And in a brief flirtation, each recognized in the other an ally, someone who could help the other get out of the dark, dead-end life each was living. Bud calls it the "Hansel and Gretel" myth. Two children lost in the deep, dark forest forged a partnership to escape.

Bud took Nellie to the theater and gave her a piece of his dream. They started dating. Bud flourished in the comfortable, accepting, low-stress relationship. In the light of Nellie's love, he could see a future outside of Norwalk. For Nellie's part, she desired a way out of the poverty and cultural straitjacket in which she was trapped. Bud was the answer.

The first ever in his family to seek a degree, Bud had enrolled at Cerritos Junior College, but the same inertia he had in high school followed him there. Then, with the advent of Nellie, they both recognized that Bud's intellect could be the vehicle to rescue them from the economic and cultural desert in which they were lost.

Bud's grades soared with his spirits. His partnership with Nellie gave him the motivation to achieve, and he completed his two years at Cerritos with academic honors. Bud and Nellie were married. Given Nellie's Lutheran background and Bud's aversion to alcohol, it was a dry wedding. As Bud and Nellie left the reception, he saw his father pouring himself a drink. Later, they heard from friends and relatives alike that their reception was the most raucous party any had been to in years. Apparently, his father offered one of Nellie's uncles a drink. He accepted. Lutherans don't drink often, but, before long, most of the relatives were imbibing, and the party lasted long into the night. One staunch cousin, infuriated at his weak relatives' sinfulness, left the reception and walked two hours to get home.

As Bud gained success, he developed an intellectual and cultural inferiority complex. He knew he had the brains and work ethic to make it out of his social prison, but felt he was entering realms in which he truly did not belong. Searching for four-year schools to complete his degree, he found many prestigious colleges courting him. During the early sixties, social egalitarianism was sweeping the country as the civil rights movement made headlines almost daily. Bud vividly remembers an interview he had at one of the Claremont colleges, renowned bastions of social and educational excellence. As he walked into the foyer of the administration building, he encountered a stunningly beautiful young lady in formal attire playing magnificently on a grand piano. It was as if the starving street urchin had watched a Christmas feast from the window. Bud was impressed, but he felt uncomfortable in such high-class company. He accepted admission at Cal State-Fullerton, a campus of the burgeoning California State College system.

Even at a state college, the mechanic's son from the blue-collar neighborhood felt increasing tension. Bud was rising well above his prior social station, and the fear of entering a forbidden intellectual province, coupled with the hard work of balancing studies with a number of part-time jobs, left Bud highly anxious. After studying at night, he could not sleep. So he began to drink.

Why would a smart young man who recognized he was out of control when he drank resort to alcohol to calm his nerves and permit sleep? It was out of perceived necessity, and one of the subtle seductions of alcohol is that he felt he could handle it. The transition from a few drinks to relax to hard-core alcoholism is so slow and subtle that it is rarely noticed. But the need was there for Bud. Ignoring the warnings of his past experience, he relied on liquor to help him cope.

At first it was beer. But the sheer volume of beer he had to drink to produce somnolence was daunting. In relatively short order, beer gave way to wine, and then wine gave way to hard liquor, as it required the smallest volume for the best and quickest effect. Each night, Bud would literally drink himself to sleep.

With his hopes combined with those of his beloved Nellie riding on his shoulders, Bud felt the burden. Sixteen-hour days of study and work ended at ten o'clock when Bud cracked the whiskey bottle open. After three stiff shots, he would tumble senseless into bed.

As any neurologist will attest, this is not restful sleep. Alcohol produces sleep by depressing the nervous system, a narcosis similar to general anesthesia greatly reducing normal brain activity. But normal brain activity is vital to healthy sleep. The brain functions in a very complex manner during sleep, cycling from states of deep restful sleep to vivid dreaming states associated with REM sleep and back again all night. Each of these sleep states, especially the REM stage, is essential to renew normal, healthy brain function. In sleep lab experiments, people who are deliberately awakened each time they approach the REM stage, effectively preventing that stage, progressively develop serious emotional disorders, which may eventuate in frank psychosis.

Unknowingly, Bud was preventing himself from getting the rest he needed. The stupor of alcohol is not the restful sleep of sobriety. The alcohol-induced sleep exacerbated the anxiety and tension in his life. Feeling tired and stressed all the time, Bud responded by drinking more.

And so it went. Bud drank his way through college at Cal State-Fullerton and on to graduate school for his PhD in history at the University of Georgia. It is a tribute to Bud's intellect and his determination that, despite his drinking, he accomplished so much. Aiding in his success was his discovery that vigorous exercise was a great stress releaser as well. Bud was a good athlete, and physical activity came easily to him. He began to run, cycle, and swim. Despite his drinking, he became extremely fit and experienced the endorphin high that is the natural reward of sustained intense physical activity. Between the exercise and the booze, Bud was just barely able to cope.

Bud couldn't escape his torment, the constant feeling he was being judged. He desperately wanted to be part of the world he aspired to, a college professor and aficionado of fine art, music, and drama. He possessed the intellect and work ethic, but the tension of feeling like an outsider was enormous. He couldn't avoid the fear that his professors and peers would discover he was the blue-collar urchin he was inside. The Impostor Syndrome is surprisingly common. Though talented and bright, he believed he was aspiring to something he didn't deserve, going someplace he had no right to be. And he was sure the guardians of the status quo would find him out and expose him for the fraud he really was.

And so Bud drank. As his tolerance increased, he began to drink during the day. As he did, his performance gradually deteriorated. And with time, as he will admit, his morality deteriorated as well. He began to hide how much he drank from Nellie and his colleagues.

It was a fifteen-year process, the insidious downward spiral of more liquor, lower-quality work, more guilt, more anxiety, and more liquor. Without realizing it, Bud had become a hard-core alcoholic. He would wake up shaky and drink to quiet the tremors. And with each passing month, it took more whiskey to calm those shakes and more whiskey to quiet those fears. It was a nightmare. He couldn't live with alcohol, and he couldn't live without it.

I saw Bud as a patient for a year or so during this terrible time. I recall smelling the strong odor of alcohol on his breath and observing intoxicated behavior, wondering if his wife knew how serious his drinking was and wondering how long he could continue with such an obvious problem.

There have been times in my practice when I observed patients coming visit after visit, clearly intoxicated. Somehow, they function drunk for years without dying of liver disease or getting arrested for drunk driving. They reach some kind of alcoholic equilibrium where their behavior, alcohol intake, and luck remain the same. This was not so with Bud. His drinking continued to increase as his life approached the brink of crisis. He drank so much that he could no longer train, losing the endorphin high that had sustained him for many years. He was at the breaking point.

Nellie was in denial about the severity of Bud's alcoholism. She knew he drank heavily, but she would not confront him because it might jeopardize their future. It was too painful to remember the menial jobs of her childhood. Bud was her white knight, who drank to cope.

On the verge of self-destruction, drinking two quarts of whiskey a day, and perhaps sensing imminent disaster, Bud went to counseling six times. At the end of the sixth visit, the therapist told Bud there was nothing wrong with him. He was simply a liar and a drunk. The therapist's comment hit Bud like a slap in the face. He could no longer deny it. He was a hopeless drunk. And he knew he was killing himself.

His therapist engineered an intervention. Bud's loved ones confronted him, and they coerced him into a treatment center in Monterey. Shortly after arrival, he developed the DTs. Suddenly withdrawn from a drug he had abused every day for the last twenty-five years, Bud was close to death. He had high fevers and cold sweats. He hallucinated. He had seizures. He was so sick that the staff suggested sending him to the local community hospital, but the center's doctor refused, convinced they were no better equipped to treat Bud's crisis than he was. They wouldn't know there existed a fine human being, a person worth salvaging, inside the pathetic and tragic figure Bud had become. The doctor won. After many long nights, the crisis passed, and Bud recovered. He spent thirty-five days in the Monterey Center and was discharged fully detoxed. He was clean and sober, but returned to the same environment with the same fears and shame, a situation portending failure. Realizing he needed some time to work out changes in his life, Bud was able to convince his department head to grant him three months of disability. He spent them at the Alano Club, learning how not to drink.

For three months, Bud went to AA meetings, sometimes three and four a day. He acknowledged his addiction, and he learned from others like him not to make excuses and rebuild a life without alcohol. This was the practical side of his recovery, the nuts and bolts of being sober. But the AA concept of "one day at a time" drove him nuts. He acknowledged the minute-to-minute decision not to drink is what would save him, but his psyche required the long view of life. He needed to see his life in terms of continuous long-lasting sobriety. He needed to better understand the complexity of his personality, the needs that had nearly driven him to oblivion. For that, he turned to therapy. For Bud, they went hand in hand. AA provided the practical solution; therapy supplied the intellectual. For sobriety, there were meetings. For sanity, there was his therapist.

Bud's keen mind began to marvel at the insights he discovered about himself, addiction, and getting healthy. The natural result was a master's degree in psychology and a license in family and marriage counseling. He gradually wound down his teaching career as his psychology practice grew. His forte, of course, is substance abuse. What better qualifications could he have than the twenty-five years of alcoholism he has lived? He knows every excuse because he's used them each more than once. He's used every rationalization imaginable, fooling almost everyone but himself. He can see through the smoke screen of BS that most alcoholics hide behind. There's no hiding from Bud. He's been there before.

If the patient has any desire to discover the truth and save himself, Bud has answers to start him on his way. He has done dozens of interventions like the one that ultimately saved him. He knows how to put the two together—the practical and the intellectual—to get the person sober, but to give insight into the personality flaws that have led to this circumstance.

He doesn't always succeed, but not from lack of knowledge and commitment. He feels his work is both an obligation and a privilege. He is grateful to be alive, and he knows that AA is not enough. Unless he can give his patient strategies for coping, insight into why the addiction occurred, and a love of the sober person he has within, he can't affect a long-term recovery. Otherwise, it's day-to-day sobriety, that is, habits without understanding. With only half the answer, the relapse rate is frightening.

When Bud got sober, he came back to see me as a patient. His honesty was disarming. Fascinated with the insights he had into the problem, I was in awe of the courage it took to do what he had done. Even then, sixteen years ago, I didn't like the control alcohol had over me. I was ashamed of my weakness, and I knew I needed alcohol too much. But I was powerless to change back then. I never let on to Bud that I had a problem. I just listened to him explain his growth through the recovery process. I listened to him describe the lives of hopelessness some of his patients endured and acknowledged by my agreement that alcohol was a huge problem for many people. But I never admitted that I was one of them.

Bud was my mentor. Once a quarter, we'd have coffee in the early morning and talk about life. We talked about spiritual growth and the challenges of being an honest person in a world that doesn't honor integrity as much as cleverness. We talked about how we could remain beacons of virtue in a sea of immorality. We agreed that, when the society that worships money and power finally self-destructs, we might be able to preserve a tiny bit of the culture and save it for the renaissance. And we were both certain that we needed each other and like-minded souls to keep the light alive. Additionally, we agreed it was enough if we could save one soul at a time. And all along, I secretly knew I couldn't be true to the righteousness that I aspired to as long as I was drinking. It was similar to discovering I couldn't run any better while I was still smoking. When running became important enough, I quit the smoking. I knew that, when the spiritual need grew great enough, I would quit drinking. But, despite the fact I had beaten other addictions (amphetamines and cigarettes), I could not find the strength within me I needed to quit. Looking back, I realize it was because I was not completely committed spiritually. I could still hold back a little and be Jeff Herten, in control of my life and my drinking. I could quit anytime I wanted. I was the boss, and I had the strength. But as the years rolled by, I was still drinking. I was not totally committed, and an emptiness was in my heart. One day, I realized I was strong, but not strong enough to quit. I needed more strength than I had. I needed a higher power. When I finally surrendered and allowed myself to be filled with that power, I couldn't drink anymore. They were diametrically opposed.

When I quit, it was a joy to tell Bud about it. Now I am completely honest with him, completely in agreement on how drinking costs a person his soul. We still have coffee together, but now there is nothing but the truth between us.

I love the person that I have become sober. I revel in the strength that it took for me to quit, and I thank God daily for that strength and saving my life.

Fortunately for me, I didn't have to drink to the brink of oblivion like Bud did to finally quit. I quit when I realized I was powerless to quit alone. That awareness made all the difference.

BUD'S INSIGHT

I asked my friend Bud why people drink. There are many reasons really: grief, sadness, depression, pain, illness, and anger. There's grief over the loss of loved ones, prostates, colons, and breasts. There's sadness that life is passing us by and so many of our dreams are unreachable. There's depression from growing older and more infirm, but no closer to the truth. There's pain, psychic and physical, and our seeming helplessness to allay or prevent it. There's illness that afflicts us without rhyme, reason, or predestination from the universe. And there's anger… intense anger. There's anger at everything and nothing. There's anger at the helplessness and hopelessness of the world. There's anger at the greed, evil, injustice, poverty, and misery that have no end, no reason, and no solution. And so we drink.

THE SOBERING TRUTH

38

CONCEALING THE PROBLEM

The neurologists were puzzled. Colin Murphy had a severe and progressive neurological disease with profound muscle weakness and loss of coordination, which had developed three months prior. Not the typical profile for multiple sclerosis or Lou Gehrig's disease, Colin was a mystery until the neurologists requested a dermatology consult. I was called. The patient had peculiar white bands extending horizontally across all of his finger and toenails. They were Mee's lines, the classical clinical picture of arsenic poisoning. I took the supervising neurologist aside and explained the diagnosis. A twenty-four-hour urine for heavy metals confirmed my suspicion. Within two weeks, Colin's wife had been arrested, and the patient was dramatically better.

It's remarkable how much a trained observer can learn from looking at the skin. I was blessed with good powers of observation and a curious nature. These skills have served me well as a clinical dermatologist. Like Mee's lines, the skin presents innumerable signs of a patient's lifestyle and general health, and it is truly a window into the individual's physical and emotional life. Something as seemingly trivial as slight bluish discoloration of the fingernails with nearly imperceptible swelling of the last digit might indicate a grave lung condition. An irregular narrowing of a hair shaft may reveal a serious eating disorder. Because of my personal history with alcohol, I am particularly sensitive to the many skin signs of alcohol abuse. Twenty percent of the adult patients in my practice reveal a significant use of, if not a problem with, alcohol.

Howard, a sixty-something semiretired educator with fair skin, sees me regularly for skin cancer problems. He likes early-morning appointments, so I see him at 7:00 AM twice a year. More often than not, he has the smell of alcohol on his breath. He has very fair skin with the crimson cheeks of his northern European heritage, and they are especially flushed when I see him for his early-morning visits. I am sure he is not aware that I can detect alcohol on his breath at seven o'clock, denoting he has already been drinking or he is still off-gassing ethanol from a serious bout of drinking the night before. Howard's wife sees me at six-month intervals as well. Her visits are in the afternoon, and I have never noted alcohol on her breath or observed any of the stigmata of alcohol abuse.

Warren, an entrepreneur in his seventies, is a big man who is also obese. He had massive swelling of his parotid glands overlying his jaw on both sides, blocking the lower half of his ears from view. He suffered hardening of the arteries from years of cigarette smoking and diabetes and high blood pressure from overindulgence in food and whiskey. Parotid swelling is a hallmark of the hard drinker. The alcohol, functioning as a sugar and contributing to the obesity, played a role in producing the diabetes as well. Warren would show up for early-morning appointments with alcohol on his breath. He recently died of the complications of diabetes and arteriosclerosis, still drinking at the end.

In her late forties, Carla is a mother of two going through a nasty divorce. She is frankly tipsy and reeking of alcohol at her early-afternoon appointment.

In his late forties, John is a disabled highway worker for the state. He has a legitimate skin condition from the stress of an overbearing and dictatorial boss, but claims the pain it causes requires prescription narcotics. He has been cited several times for attempting to fill the same prescription twice before refills were needed. He also prefers early-morning appointments, and he has the smell of alcohol on his breath.

Larry is a businessman in his mid-fifties who struggles to satisfy a high-maintenance wife. During the last five years, I have noticed the capillaries on his face becoming more livid and the puffiness around his eyes more prominent. Larry drinks too much.

Dorothy was a hard-core alcoholic. Over the last ten years, I watched as her skin became more sallow, and she developed the large spider hemangiomas that indicate impending liver failure. Next, her belly grew big as an enlarged, alcoholic liver protruded beneath her rib cage. Then the liver shrank as it scarred, and the big belly was caused by ascites, a fluid that weeps from the scarred and failing liver and builds up in the abdomen. The last time I saw Dorothy, she had a coarse tremor that may have been a liver flap, another sign of impending failure as ammonia, usually detoxified by the liver, builds up in the bloodstream and the brain. She had one gastrointestinal bleed from alcoholic gastritis, and her doctor warned her that she had to stop drinking or it would kill her. It did when her liver and kidneys failed. The mortality rate of this condition, hepatorenal syndrome, is extremely high.

In medical school, students are taught to do a thorough history and physical examination. The history is a multipart record of the present illness, family history, past illnesses and surgeries, medications, review of all the systems, and a social history. Important facts in this section are marital status, job, children, and use of tobacco, alcohol, and social drugs such as marijuana, cocaine, heroin, and so on.

Because insurance companies, attorneys, and law enforcement can request these medical records, you can imagine that some of the responses to the latter questions may be less than completely candid.

As a medical student, I was taught that whatever quantity of alcohol consumption a patient admits to, the truth is probably twice that or more. If the patient says he drinks two beers a night, it is probably four or five. If he admits to two glasses of wine with dinner, he and his wife probably polish off a bottle together. People are generally embarrassed to admit how much they drink, so they naturally decrease the true amount. There are obvious exceptions. People who totally abstain are often vehement about it, and they can be trusted. Some alcoholics completely deny imbibing, but the evidence of their dishonesty is displayed all over their bodies. With time, a clever interviewer can spot the inconsistency between the history and physical findings.

On the other hand, some heavy drinkers and frank alcoholics are quite honest about how much they drink. They will candidly report that they drink a twelve-pack of beer or more a night, a fifth of bourbon, or a bottle-

and-a-half of wine. Some are curiously proud of their accomplishment. Recovering alcoholics are usually quite honest about their past abuse, and it is astonishing to learn how much a person can drink and not die, at least in the short term.

Doctors use cryptic shorthand to identify the drinking habits of their patients. It developed long before there was concern that medical records were discoverable by attorneys and might end up in court, that is, before all the current concern about the privacy of a patient's medical record. It was just a coded way for the physician to record his observations in the patient's chart without it being obvious to someone other than another doctor.

Interesting notations show up in the margin or the text of the chart note for that visit. "HBD" in the margin of the chart stood for "has been drinking." "ETOH" was a less subtle notation, representing an abbreviation for ethanol, the chemical name for ethyl alcohol. Another surreptitious way of documenting such observations would be to write "twocarbon disease," as alcohol is a two-carbon molecule. "2-C problem" is another and perhaps even more obscure way to record the obvious signs of alcoholism in a patient without creating an easily understandable note for the office staff or insurance claims person who might read the patient's chart.

In recent years, some of my colleagues have become less charitable. On the problem list heading the patient's chart is "Problem 3: Alcohol abuse." Bear in mind that the American Psychiatric Association defines alcohol abuse as drinking one or more drinks three times a week. That doesn't leave many out, does it? I often wondered how plaintiffs' attorneys handle these chart note entries in court. Say the patient is suing for complications that occurred after a surgery, perhaps a wound infection. The notation of "alcohol abuse" is a social stigma for the patient, and the common medical knowledge that alcohol suppresses the immune system and increases the potential for infection would make pursuing this suit difficult at best, especially before a jury.

As a young physician, I never felt comfortable frankly confronting patients' alcohol habits. I observed and recorded the progressive signs of liver damage and failure on Dorothy's chart, but I never mentioned it to her. I was somewhat embarrassed to bring it up and partly, as an HFA, I felt I didn't have the right to judge my patients. Now sober, I still try not to judge my alcoholic patients because I see alcohol addiction as a disease and not a character disorder, but I try to help patients become aware they have a bigger problem than they realize.

Last week, Tom, a businessman in his mid-forties, was in the office for an exam. He had all the signs of heavy drinking, puffiness around the eyes; coarse, dilated capillaries over his nose; a fine tremor; and several new spiders on his face and upper back. I have noticed alcohol on his breath several times in past visits. Not all spiders are signs of severe liver problems. They occur normally in fair-skinned people, young adolescent females on oral contraceptives, and pregnant women. But adding it all up, I decided that perhaps Tom needed to know that his alcoholism was taking a toll. I pointed out one of the spiders and asked how long it had been there.

"Six months," he responded. "What caused them?"

"Well, sometimes they just happen. At other times, they may be an indication of internal problems."

"What kind of internal problems?"

"Well, I am sure this doesn't apply to you, but sometimes they are the sign of early liver damage from drinking. But you don't drink that much, do you?"

"Not that much. I drink a couple of beers a night."

Translated, this is at least a six-pack. His concern is way out of proportion for someone who really drinks two beers a night.

"That's not enough to cause spiders," I said. "Sometimes, these just occur in fair-skinned people, and that's probably the answer."

He wouldn't let it go. "How does drinking cause spiders?"

Again, I assured him that this couldn't apply to him, but explained that, in heavy drinkers, the damaged liver can't break down estrogens and higher levels of circulating estrogens cause the spiders.

"But don't worry," I said. "If it were really from liver damage, you'd notice other things."

"Like what?"

"Well, the increased estrogen causes the testicles to shrivel up. Makes you impotent."

I watched his pupils get large. It was obvious I had his attention.

"You don't have any problems like that?"

"No," he lied.

The greatest shame for a man is not functioning sexually, so I'm not surprised he denied it. The look of concern was written on his face. I had scored a direct hit, but he tried not to let on.

"Is there any way to treat or repair the liver damage?"

"It's pretty far advanced at that point, but the liver is an amazingly resilient organ, and some repair is possible if the drinker abstains."

We ended the visit with Tom still trying to ask questions and with me reassuring him that couldn't be the problem by his drinking history. Tom is a hypochondriac. Perhaps his anxiety over health concerns will force him to face his alcohol problem. I had been honest with him. Perhaps I had an impact.

Physicians sometimes make critical errors in not realizing how heavily their patients drink. A well-respected judge who alleges to drinking a glass of wine at dinner had an abnormal liver function test. This prompted the physician to do an expensive and fruitless workup for hepatitis and rare liver diseases when the problem is that the judge drinks too much. I saw a case recently of a prominent local businessman who repeatedly had elevated liver enzymes. The clinician did an exhaustive workup and found nothing, yet, every time he checked the patient's blood, those same liver enzymes were elevated. As a result, the doctor scheduled a liver biopsy, not the most benign procedure. A long, large gauge needle is inserted in the patient's right midback, aiming for the liver. Done correctly, a small core sample of liver is recovered. With poor or unlucky aim, a large artery in the liver might be punctured or lacerated, causing massive bleeding.

Occasionally, the lower edge of the chest cavity is penetrated, and the patient suffers a pneumothorax (punctured lung). As a pathology resident, I interpreted liver biopsies. Occasionally, a piece of kidney was all that was recovered from the needle. Suffice it to say, a liver biopsy is not an entirely safe procedure. I treat patients with psoriasis with a medication that is toxic to the liver, and periodic liver biopsies are mandatory to ensure the patient is not progressing to cirrhosis. When I request one, the gastroenterologist always makes me insist I really need it because he doesn't like performing them. So this really high-risk biopsy is being done on a patient to assess his liver when the real problem is that he drinks a liter of wine every night. But the judge and his doctor never had an honest conversation about how much he was really drinking, nor did the doctor insist he abstain for a week or two before repeating the liver enzymes. Knowing both the doctor and patient well, I was astounded they had never had that conversation. Before I submit my patient to a liver biopsy, I certainly would.

With hard-core alcoholics, information and education about the progression of their liver disease does no good. They are out of control and literally unable to stop once they start drinking until they pass out. But they have heard the words. They know the negative consequences of their addiction.

There is a saying among recovering alcoholics, "The alcoholic is the last one to know." It's true. The wife knows, the boss knows, coworkers know, the children know, and friends know. The trash man who empties five empty vodka bottles a week knows. The doctor knows. But cunning, baffling, powerful alcohol masks the truth from the drinker until the very end. Then the inexorable progression of the disease takes its toll.

THE SOBERING TRUTH

39

THE DRUNK IN THE BOARDROOM

When I was growing up, my parents had a large and interesting circle of friends. Many factors bound them together. The women belonged to several volunteer organizations. Most of the group played golf, and all were upper middle class. To a person, they all drank.

Jack McDougall, a member of the group, fascinated me. An enormously successful realtor, Jack was chairman of the board of the second-largest real estate firm in the nation. He took it public when I was in my twenties, realizing tens of millions of dollars in stock. But if you met Jack at a barbecue or party, you'd never guess he was a shrewd, successful businessman. He looked, talked, and drank like an old cowboy.

Jack grew up in McKittrick, California, a bleak, little town on the western side of the San Joaquin Valley, most notable for its large deposits of oil. He grew up riding horses and doing hard physical work, went to UC-Berkeley, worked for a time for the IRS, and then found that his Will Rogers persona and financial aspirations were ideal for the real estate business. What's more, in all his endeavors, Jack found he had a secret weapon, an advantage over his clients and the competition. Jack McDougall could drink vast quantities and function at a very high level.

To enhance his image, Jack rolled his own cigarettes, a throwback to his old wrangler days. It was enthralling to watch him pull a little cloth sack of tobacco out of his shirt pocket, pour it with one hand onto a cigarette paper, close the purse string of the pouch with his teeth, curl the paper to concentrate the tobacco, lick the edge, and expertly roll a stubby but firm cigarette.

I would watch Jack with fascination when he came to our home for a dinner party. Before dinner, he matched my dad drink for drink. This warm-up consisted of two or three hard liquor drinks. With dinner, there was wine. With dessert, they drank Kahlua, Galliano, or brandy. Then, when the party stretched into the wee hours, Jack would switch to beer. Looking back, I am astounded at the volume of alcohol that was consumed. Jack's consumption equaled anyone's, but I never saw him drunk. He would just stand there with his shoulders set at a confident angle, cigarette in his left hand, his right hand gesturing to make a point, and clear and observant eyes accenting his weather-beaten face. A very smart man, he exuded a quiet confidence, but never arrogance.

Jack McDougall knew how to use that intelligence, his very personable social skills, and his ability to drink to rise to the top of the real estate business. He was as comfortable in the locker rooms of the most exclusive country clubs as he was on a horse. At work, Jack kept a fifth of bourbon and several glasses on the sideboard in his office. It was his secretary's responsibility to replace it with a full one daily. And each day, usually with some help from clients and business partners, that bottle would be empty by quitting time. Negotiations were undertaken over a drink. Contracts were signed and deals were sealed with a handshake and a drink. And when the bargaining got tense and heated, the coolest man in the room, with the highest blood alcohol level, was Jack McDougall. How many bargains did he strike intoxicated? How many concessions and compromises did he gain because he was able to hold his liquor better than his adversary? Lots.

Jack once told me that he only did business two days a week: Tuesday and Thursday. When I looked startled, he explained.

"Jeff, you never try to make a deal on Monday. Your customer just got back from a weekend at the lake, and his mind is still there. On Wednesday, he plays golf in the afternoon, so his mind isn't on business in the morning. On Friday, he's getting ready to go away for the weekend, and his mind is already there. So you never call him those days. Tuesdays and Thursdays, that's when I do all my business."

Of course, he was right. Jack figured it all out early in his career and used it to his advantage. In his later years, Jack's cancerous larynx was removed. He used a small handheld silver amplifier to squawk out short responses. Mouth and throat cancer have two major predisposing factors: tobacco and alcohol. The doctors at his alma mater were miraculously able to save him, and he lived to a ripe age, into his late eighties, croaking with his silver amplifier and smiling that wry smile.

I can imagine you're wondering, "What's wrong with the way he lived? He was fabulously successful and respected in the business community, and he had raised a family, enjoyed life, and lived into old age. What's wrong with that?"

The answer is nothing, if you agree that Jack McDougall alone did not do all those things. It wasn't Jack who made the money, raised those kids, and enjoyed those rodeos. It was Jack and alcohol. It was Jack fortified with whiskey.

So what? So alcohol was a crutch, a coping mechanism, and a tool Jack McDougall used to function successfully in his world. It calmed his nerves while he negotiated the big deals and eased his social anxiety at big board meetings. It gave him that competitive edge working in the world of high finance. It made him feel good.

What if his drug of choice had been heroin? What if it had been crack cocaine or crystal meth? Would that have been okay? Why is one drug, alcohol, socially acceptable and another, heroin, not? Why is the person addicted to cocaine treated as a pariah, while the person addicted to alcohol is revered and emulated? Is it because alcohol is legal? There is a disconnect here in our social consciousness. If Jack had landed in the gutter, his alcoholism may have been viewed as a problem. In the plush boardrooms of the Fortune 500, it is not. Why not? Alcohol, although legal, is a drug, and Jack is an addict.

We're not arguing over whether Jack McDougall was a drug addict or not. He was. We're just arguing that the drug he became addicted to does not carry the social stigma of heroin or crack cocaine.

The important point is that Jack didn't need alcohol to climb the ladder of success. If he could do it drunk, he could do it better sober. He had the right stuff in him. He just didn't think he could. When deprived of their chemical coping mechanism, some people are convinced they can't function. In truth, they can and will function as well or better if they find strength elsewhere in their lives.

THE SOBERING TRUTH

# ERNEST HEMINGWAY

He could say more with fewer words than any other author. He captured the beauty and emotion of a scene like few others I have ever read. As a young writer, he'd spend days honing a two-page description of a scene into a single paragraph. He said that what you left out was more important than what you put in. When reading his novels, one has to imagine his intent at times. These mysterious omissions make his writing so engaging. Ernest Hemingway, Nobel Prize winner and one of the greatest writers of the twentieth century, struggled with alcoholism all his life, and it coauthored his demise.

He was born into the upper middle class in a wealthy suburb of Chicago, the son of a doctor who committed suicide at an early age. As a boy, Hemingway spent his summers in the Upper Peninsula of Michigan, leaving him with a lifelong love of fishing, hunting, and the rugged self-reliance of the outdoorsman. He left his home and country to drive an ambulance in Italy in World War I and then lived in Paris, joining a group of self-exiled American artists that included Ezra Pound and Gertrude Stein. And he wrote. And he drank.

Hemingway was obsessed with masculinity. He boxed, wrestled, brawled, hunted, fished, and drank with gusto. He fancied himself a great lover, but, by all accounts, he was mediocre. Being rather self-absorbed, it is unlikely that he was interested in pleasuring a partner or he was sober enough to do so most of the time.

Hemingway suffered black periods when he couldn't create and drank hard. As he matured, he began to realize that he couldn't drink and write. He would go on the wagon, rise early, write for three or four hours, and rediscover his creative genius. He was physically healthy, lived a Spartan life, and wrote well and prolifically. Some of his greatest literary achievements were accomplished during these periods. Hemingway was always content during these times of creativity and sobriety. Inevitably, however, upon completion of a book, he would begin drinking hard again.

As the years passed and his fame grew, so did the friends and hangers-on. Solitude, discipline, and sobriety were harder to achieve. Celebrity brought wealth and more opportunities to travel, hunt, party, and drink. As a result, he began to have difficulty with high blood pressure. The alcoholic calories that expanded his waistline exacerbated his blood pressure problem. The physical deterioration caused by his alcoholism—high blood pressure, failing eyesight, memory loss, poor concentration, and lack of endurance, strength, and sexual prowess—caused severe depression.

During the last decade of his life as an aging writer, the Nobel Prize and lucrative movie contracts in hand, he struggled to create for a demanding public. But his physical and mental decline rendered him incapable of his previous genius. He suffered intractable hypertension and obsessively took his blood pressure, logging it in a small book dozens of times a day. Robbed of his discipline and gift of prose, his inability to cope created a psychotic depression. The delicate balance of neurotransmitters that determines state of mind had gone tragically awry, in part abetted by years of alcoholism.

And as is so common in the progression of alcoholism, the drinking that had always been able to soothe the depression now magnified it, leading to a failed suicide attempt. The pain had grown too great. There was no hope of regaining his creative genius. Suicide was Hemingway's only solution. One autumn day in Idaho, he put the barrel of a shotgun in his mouth and definitively ended his agony.

The scene is not uncommon, great minds with sacred gifts squandered in a losing battle with alcohol addiction. We need to make the public more aware that alcohol brings wildly exciting abandonment to pleasure and lack of inhibition, but it also comes with a yoke of dependence that, for many, is difficult or impossible to shed. The short-term glamour, excitement, and sexiness of alcohol may be replaced with physical and psychological addiction and a depression that few are able to tolerate. With the immersion of our culture in the media blitz created by the alcohol industry, this is a daunting challenge. Perhaps by telling our stories and those tragedies like Ernest Hemingway's, we can open eyes and minds to the peril.

THE SOBERING TRUTH

41

ALCOHOLISM & AA

Discipline is my middle name. I'm the guy who never missed a day of running in two years, the guy who got up at 4:30 every morning so I could get ten miles in before work, worked a full day, and then ran five miles after work for months at a time. I quit nail biting. I quit cigarettes. I quit amphetamines. I lost thirty-five pounds on the Atkins diet. Yes, sir, I have a will of iron. I could will myself to run the last seventy-five miles of a hundred-mile run with a sprained ankle.

Quit drinking? No problem. I'd quit so many times that I'd lost count. But there was just one problem. I couldn't maintain it. I'd always start again. Then one day, shamed and humiliated, I wanted to quit more than I ever wanted anything in my life. But I knew I was powerless to do it on my own. So I got down on my knees and asked my higher power to take this burden, this addiction, off my shoulders. And he did. He did what I couldn't do. He led me to sobriety. And as long as I remember that it is through his grace and love that I got sober, through his power and not my own, I can stay sober.

One of the remarkable ironies of alcoholism is that willpower and personal strength often fail in the end. The proud alcoholic, who, like me, truly believes he can quit anytime he wills it, is sadly deluded. Personal strength is a real handicap in the quest for sobriety. It takes years for an arrogant alcoholic like me to come to the awareness that he has a problem, then years more for him to realize that he can't fix it himself. By then, he has lost a job, a wife, or both. Perhaps he's had a couple of

DUIs or hurt someone while driving under the influence. He's lost his temper in a drunken rage and screamed at his children so many times that it's now a learned response in them, and they're likely to treat their kids similarly. Oftentimes, the proud and arrogant person never gets it. He never realizes that alcohol is too "cunning, baffling, and powerful" (Alcoholics Anonymous 2001) to overcome alone. A rare individual is strong enough to achieve sobriety without help from a higher power.

Personal strength alone is not the answer. It didn't work for my friend Kate. She grew up in an alcoholic family and started drinking after she was raped at the age of thirteen. She stole most of her booze by walking into a liquor store and walking out with a fifth of tequila when the clerk was occupied with another customer. No one would suspect a cute thirteen-year-old girl.

Kate drank hard until she was thirty-five. Then, after a near-crippling accident, she experienced a moment of clarity that allowed her to see what a mess her life was and how it had all started with alcohol. She quit the same day, summoning all of her personal strength and discarding every bottle she had in the house.

But Kate didn't seek support to stay sober. She figured she could do it on her own. She didn't get professional help, join AA, and begin the process of identifying the issues that had led her to drink. She was sober, but not seeking the understanding and contentment that could keep her sober.

She lasted a little over a year. I planned to relate her experience in detail, but, when I sent a draft of her chapter, she fired back a terse note that she didn't want to bare herself, share her story. I wrote back, inquiring if she were still sober. There was no reply.

It happens. Alcoholics fall off the wagon, even those who ask their higher power to take over for them. But it happens a lot more often to the alcoholic who fights his addiction alone. He just doesn't have the ammunition to battle such a formidable foe.

Strong-willed sober alcoholics who don't seek support risk becoming dry drunks. They still have the problems, bad temper, dishonesty, and feelings of guilt and inferiority they had when drinking. They are sober, yet sobriety has not provided them peace and contentment. Some obsess about alcohol more than when they were drinking. I heard a fellow say that, for the three years he was sober, he couldn't get through a day without thinking about alcohol. Finally, when he began drinking again, he had a tremendous sense of relief. He was drinking instead of obsessing about it. He drank for a year before his life became so unmanageable that he accepted rehab again and acknowledged for the first time that he couldn't do it by himself. He surrendered to alcohol. He gave up trying to win a battle that he now knew he could not win alone. Strategic surrender is the road that leads to sobriety and happiness.

Sally's worried face reflected that her son, Rick, was in jail again. It was another DUI. He had just gotten his license back after two years.

"I know he'll quit this time. He's a very strong person. If they threaten to put his son in a foster home, I know he can quit."

Probably not. Rick will quit when he realizes that alcohol is ruining his life and he can't quit on his own, but needs support to fight this battle. But Rick is proud, and he may not get it this time. Surrender takes humility.

Pride and a sense of personal strength also lead many alcoholics to believe they can drink moderately. They want to be social drinkers like other people. The goal of drinking like a gentleman has them drinking just at parties on the weekends for a while. But fairly quickly, they are drinking almost every day. Sooner rather than later, their lives are out of control again.

What if you don't believe in a higher power? You're unsure that there is a God, so how can you call on Him for help? When you are desperate enough, when you have been humbled and humiliated enough to realize you can't do it alone, simply ask. It requires a rigorous honesty to finally have that moment of truth, to know there really is no other way. That awareness is truly an unrealized gift. He is asking you to let Him help. Suppress your ego and pride, and ask for His help. Ask Him to lift this crushing burden from your shoulders. You may be shocked at the results.

I was. The dark night of hopeless futility suddenly became a brilliant dawn of freedom. It was a miracle, an incredible gift of grace that proved to me there was a higher power. It proved to me that He loved me and He wanted me sober. For that, I thank Him daily.

THE SOBERING TRUTH

42

LESSONS FROM THE LIBERTY TATTOO CLINIC

The brilliant, rapid-fire yellow flares light the wall behind me. The sound resembles a muffled automatic weapon. The black swastika on Chuck's upper arm disappears four millimeters at a time as the skin frosts white beneath the pulses of laser light. The beam sweeps up and down his tattoo, each pulse removing a tiny bit of hate. Glistening beads of sweat swell on Chuck's forehead as, teeth clenched, he bears the pain. Hunched over, holding his arm, I breathe slow and steady, trying to keep the goggles from fogging over my mask. In several minutes, it is done, the faint red of hemorrhage spreading from the edge of the treated area. Expertly, the wound is covered with aloe vera gel, a gauze pad, and a roll of gauze wrapped securely around the arm to hold it in place.

Chuck is a heavy equipment operator. He is six-foot-six and a solid two hundred and forty pounds with arms like an NFL lineman. In a prior life, he was the enforcer in a white supremacist prison gang, and his appearance is intimidating.

"Doc, I can't thank you enough for what you're doing," he says meekly.

"You're thanking me by staying clean and doing your part to save a few more like you, Chuck."

"Oh, don't worry, Doc. I'm never going down that road again. That road's for losers."

"See you in a couple months, Chuck."

"You got it, Doc."

This was Chuck's third treatment. At the first, he was stiff and self-conscious, but now he was clearly at ease and friendly. He spent six years in prison for armed robbery because of his addiction to methamphetamine and alcohol. His arms were free of the needle marks and scars of some of my heroin addict patients, but menacing tattoos covered them.

Slowly, these remnants of his former life were disappearing beneath the flashing beam of our Q-switched neodynium-yttrium-argon-gallium laser (Nd-YAG). The intense laser light, delivered in pulses of a millionth of a second, is absorbed by the small pigment granules that constitute the tattoo. The light is converted to heat and vibration, breaking the granules into small enough pieces for the body to digest. A layer of pigment disappears under the flashing light of the Nd-YAG laser.

Chuck is one of a hundred and fifty patients that I am treating in the Liberty clinic, which offers tattoo removal in return for community service. It is open to anyone with tattoos that are socially offensive or dangerous or prevent people from obtaining employment or advancing beyond a menial position at their job.

My work at Liberty has been a real education. Three-quarters of my patients are recovering drug and alcohol abusers. Many have been in prison. Most have been as low as human beings can go. Nearly all of them have made a choice to clean up their lives and regain their self-respect. What a remarkable group of friendly, enthusiastic, grateful, and honest people. It is powerful to learn their stories and help them rebuild their lives. They all possess a quiet dignity that results from fighting their nearly hopeless battles against alcohol and drugs. And they candidly share their stories with each other and me. They have taught me a great deal.

The first and most telling fact I learned is that alcohol was the first step in every one of their descents into addiction. For every heroin addict and meth head, the journey started with alcohol.

Second, at the height of their abuse, alcohol remained a mainstay of their addictive behavior. For each, it was drug X and alcohol. If the drug of choice wasn't available because of supply issues or lack of funds, alcohol was always there, cheap and accessible, to maintain mental oblivion until the next big score. To a person, these recovering addicts don't differentiate between cocaine, liquor, crystal meth, or heroin. It is all the same disease to them. It's not as if they graduated from alcohol to heroin. They just added the heroin to the alcohol.

A review of a few case studies from Liberty will highlight the effect of alcohol. Chuck, one of my more recent patients, grew up in a blue-collar area of Los Angeles. His father was an alcoholic who beat Chuck and his mother with regularity at night. He was never sober. By the time he was thirteen, Chuck made it a point to be out with his friends at night. He didn't come home until late, when his father had passed out or gone to sleep in an alcoholic stupor. His junior high school friends were all white in a neighborhood with many Hispanics and a few Asians and blacks. In a racial minority, these whites banded together.

Chuck started drinking occasionally when he was ten and regularly when he was thirteen. He joined a white supremacist gang avowed to eliminate all nonwhites from their turf. Its members ranged in age from thirteen to fifty, so buying alcohol was not a problem. Recreational activities included ingesting alcohol, smoking marijuana, taking speed, riding motorcycles, and sharing women.

The gang had graduates in prison and alumni in cemeteries, the victims of gang violence or motorcycling under the influence. Ironically, I had worked in an emergency room in my residency and met one of them. One of the most horrific injuries I ever dealt with was a senior member of Chuck's gang who, drunk and high on methamphetamine, put his mama on the back of his Harley and rode it down the street at three o'clock in the morning with no headlights. Lack of headlights was his first mistake; riding the wrong way on a one-way street was his second. A car hit him and his girlfriend head-on. The woman was dead at the scene. The rider was folded in half, backward under the car. When he arrived in my emergency room, he was still alive, barely. His head had been crushed on one side so it looked like he had two disparate halves stuck together, and he was in profound shock. I started large IVs and ran in massive amounts of fluid as I rode with him to the trauma center for treatment, but, mercifully, he succumbed on the way.

Growing up, Chuck never knew a high school graduate. His compadres either had been arrested or dropped out to go to work before they graduated. Needing money for drugs and alcohol, he held up a convenience store, and he was then arrested. It wasn't his first. They gave him five to ten, and he served six. Life in prison was a racial survival of the fittest. Chuck did what was necessary in order to survive, but, along the way, he realized there was no future in his present life. He joined AA and Narcotics Anonymous (NA). When released, he was fortunate enough to get a job running a backhoe for a contractor who, like him, was a recovering alcoholic and addict. Now he was married with two young children. It was hard to believe Chuck had such a sordid previous life. The tattoos attested to it, but they would soon be gone.

Sally is one of my long-standing laser patients. She has two small remnants of her five tattoos, which will require only a couple more treatments. During her former life as a biker mama, Sally was an alcoholic and drug addict. While her addiction ran the entire pharmacological gamut from meth to coke and finally to heroin, a period of several years is just a blur in her memory. She did whatever was necessary to get her drugs, often serving as the sexual slave of a dealer. But Sally is adamant that her addiction was never just heroin. It was always alcohol and heroin. She has been clean and sober for fifteen years, and the strength of her commitment to recovery is impressive. Otherwise, she'd be dead by now.

Drug addicts live a life of deadly risk. The first and foremost risk is the purity of the drug. Can you imagine buying a substance that you are going to eat or smoke, let alone inject in your veins, from a person you don't know or trust and are certain would kill you if you missed a payment? This is the addict's world. How do you know the crystal meth is pure? What is it cut with? How strong is the heroin? One of the more common scenarios in heroin addiction is death from overdose, as every batch is of a different potency. The same dose you shot up last time may kill you this time, or it may have little or no effect. One of the heroin ODs I treated while running the overdose ward at LA County-USC Hospital was brought up as a red blanket. He was comatose and barely breathing, and he had pinpoint pupils, a sure sign of heroin intoxication. He was very well dressed, and something was strikingly familiar about him. As I drew up the Narcan (the antidote to heroin), I studied his face. Then it hit me. He was an actor, star of my favorite TV western. I gave him the Narcan.

Within several minutes, he was wide-awake, embarrassed, and ashamed. He had been attending a party at another celebrity's home in the Malibu Colony. Everyone had been drinking pretty heavily when a close female friend suggested they try some heroin. He had tried it several times before with pleasant results. Wanting to please her, he said yes. She injected him, and that's the last he remembered until he awakened, looking up at a fresh-faced intern in a white jacket. If the heroin had been a little more potent, he would have died of respiratory arrest. He was lucky someone was aware enough to call 9-1-1, the paramedics responded so quickly, and the emergency medical system worked so well. For most addicts, that would not have been the case. Liberty's recovering addicts have lost several friends to overdoses.

THE SOBERING TRUTH

43

ENABLING

Nancy is one of the nicest people you'd ever want to meet. In her mid-sixties and athletic-looking, Nancy has run a number of fifty-kilometer and fifty-mile ultramarathons, winning her age group on several occasions and setting records along the way. Kind, soft-spoken, an excellent cook, and a hard worker, Nancy is a pleasure to be around. So why does this remarkable woman choose to live with hopeless alcoholics?

She lost her first husband to alcoholism. By all accounts, Ron was abusive, yet she remained with him. Totally lost in his addiction, Ron was sitting at a bar one evening with Nancy at his side when he suddenly fell backward onto the floor, dead. The cumulative effect of thirty years of hard drinking combined to scar his liver and weaken his heart. Insidiously, fluid began to back up in his lungs from a heart poisoned by alcohol. The cough that had worsened in the preceding week wasn't a virus. It was fluid filling the alveoli (air sacs) throughout his lungs. It's kind of like drowning from the inside. When nearly half the lungs are flooded, there is not enough surface area to absorb oxygen. The blood oxygen plummets, and, at some critical level, the myocardium or heart muscle, already weakened from the toxic effect of high blood alcohol levels, suddenly misfires and goes into a fatal ventricular fibrillation. Ron was dead before he hit the floor.

Within eighteen months, Nancy had met and married Larry, another alcoholic. Larry was less abusive, although he could be incredibly demeaning when he drank. Larry functioned at a remarkably high level.

A utility company employed him for thirty years. He trained countless hours on a bicycle. He had bought property, and he was building a beautiful house in the foothills of the north county. But he was drunk every day.

What is it about a person like Nancy that would make her enter into another relationship with an alcoholic? Nancy drinks, but not every day. I've never seen her drunk. She is always sober enough to drive Larry home from a barbecue. So why does she do it? Nancy is codependent. There is something about the relationship that she needs or wants, or she wouldn't stay in it. What does she want? In my experience, there are three types of people who choose to stay in relationships like Nancy's:

- The first is the classic enabler, a person who facilitates the life and activities of the alcoholic because she needs him to complete her identity. The concept is a little difficult to grasp, but the Greek myth of Narcissus and Echo best explains it. Narcissus was a lesser god who was quite handsome and enjoyed admiring himself, to the exclusion of anyone around him. Echo, a wood nymph, was madly in love with Narcissus, but the goddess Hera had cursed her for being too talkative. She could only speak in response to someone conversing with her. Echo's opportunity to speak with Narcissus soon occurred, but he spurned her. As a result, the goddess Nemesis caused Narcissus to fall hopelessly in love with his reflection in a pool of water. Thus the myth describes a critical symbiosis between a self-absorbed person oblivious to those around him and another who has no voice, or identity, except as an echo or extension of the first. Narcissus, a person so self-involved that he is concerned only with himself and his own welfare, parallels closely the alcoholic. Echo is the person with low self-esteem who does not feel she is a complete personality without the alcoholic. Echo does not feel she exists without the dominant selfish personality of Narcissus. Echo has a huge stake in ensuring that Narcissus is able to function because she is dependent on him for her survival. So, even though Narcissus is drunk most of the time, Echo enables him to pursue his alcoholism by handling the everyday details of his life. So we have Echo doing all she can to enable Narcissus to function better, even though he is a hopeless drunk. That's Nancy. She is the prototype enabler. She has accepted Larry's drinking and made allowances for it in her life. In return for her tacit acceptance, she gets the security of a nice house, a pension, a body to interact with (although frequently drunk), and a fair amount of control and decision-making in the relationship. It seems a contradiction that Nancy would have any control in the relationship. She is the quiet one, always in the background. She allows Larry to be loud, drunk, and apparently dominant. But because Larry is frequently drunk, he abdicates much of the decision-making in the relationship. He yields much of the power by virtue of the fact that he isn't functioning rationally a portion of the time. Additionally, Larry experiences some guilt, although never articulated, giving Nancy the upper hand. As an enabler, Nancy claims most of the power and shoulders only half the responsibility. She enjoys the creature comforts and companionship. For her, it is not such a bad deal. When you analyze the dynamics of the alcoholic, codependent relationship, it is much easier to understand why someone would remain. In the end, however, it all unravels, like Nancy's first marriage did when Ron died. Odds are that alcohol will kill her second husband as well.

- The second personality type that coexists with the alcoholic is a very controlling person who uses the alcohol to usurp the power in the relationship. Margaret was like that. She came from substantial wealth, and she was used to having her own way. She married Phil, a genuine war hero, after he was discharged in 1945. As they raised their family in the San Joaquin Valley, Phil's drinking progressively worsened. Margaret did nothing to intervene. On the contrary, she used the fact that he was drunk much of the time to become the dominant force in the family and relationship. Phil abdicated his role as head of the household, which she gladly assumed. This continued until they retired to the central coast. Phil got a couple DUIs, and the court mandated he go to AA. He got sober twice, but he relapsed both times. Margaret was secretly happy because his sobriety threatened the balance of power in the relationship. She liked him hopeless and dependent on her. She had not anticipated the possibility, however, that a defeated Phil would commit suicide and end the relationship for good. Amazingly, within a year, Margaret had met and married another alcoholic and set up a new fiefdom with him.

- The last type of enabler is the individual who is in total denial of the alcoholic's problem. Betty is like that. Her twenty-five-year-old son, Eric, has had three DUIs in the last year. He has been fired from his job, and the county put his three-year-old son in a foster home. He got another DUI last week. Betty was outraged. "It wasn't fair. He wasn't really drunk. He'd just had a couple beers, and he was driving home, but the registration on his car had expired, and he was pulled over." I asked what his blood alcohol level was. "He blew a 0.12 percent, but that's not really very high. He'd just had a couple beers." Betty doesn't get it. She is blind to the truth that Eric is an alcoholic and he can't drink at all, not even a couple beers! By failing to acknowledge his problem, she is enabling his alcoholism. Betty tries to shield her son from the natural consequences of his alcoholic behavior, which is simply postponing the inevitable. Bob and JoAnn Williams, aging seniors, demonstrate another example of enabling. Their daughter, Sally, is a hopeless alcoholic. When her husband left and took the kids after eight dismal, drunken years of marriage, Sally's parents bought her a condo. They give her an allowance so she can survive and drink without having to worry about work. Now in their eighties, they are arranging a trust to provide for Sally after their deaths. They are resigned to the fact that Sally is a chronic alcoholic and have made it possible for her to continue her alcoholism without adverse consequences after they are gone. Most would see the flawed logic, but the Williams think they are doing the right thing.

THE SOBERING TRUTH

44

ALCOHOLISM: CRITERIA

It's time to get personal. Most likely, you are reading this book because of your interest in alcoholism from an intimate perspective. Perhaps you suspect you are living with an alcoholic, or maybe you know you have a problem but don't know what to do. Good for you and for having the courage to look for help! The good news is that 30 percent of recovering alcoholics stay sober forever. But, in order to do so, you or your loved one has to realize and accept that there is a problem and make the commitment to change.

Are you an alcoholic? You already know, whether or not you will admit it. It's a very difficult thing to say. That's why the AA route may not initially be for everyone. It wasn't for me. Standing up in front of a group of people and saying, "My name's Jeff, and I'm an alcoholic" was something I wasn't able to do at first. Was it pride? No, it was shame. I was raised in an environment that equated actions with value. If you did something bad, you were a bad person. Shame and guilt controlled and shaped my behavior and actions while I was growing up. It has taken decades of reading, prayer, and personal growth to come to the awareness that good people can do bad things and still remain good people. We are all human and, at times, subject to human weakness. We are individually and collectively capable of messing up, and we do so quite regularly. It doesn't change our essential goodness, but it does require we acknowledge our actions, feel sincerely sorry for them, and work to avoid similar mistakes in the future. We must believe in forgiveness for ourselves, and we need to practice it with others. Truly forgiven, we are free from the burden of our mistakes and the shame and guilt that attend them. This simple awareness has been so liberating that it has changed my life. But it didn't change me enough in the beginning to make me want to proclaim my sins in front of a group of strangers. I had to find another way. This may be true as well for you or your loved one.

Back to the question. Are you an alcoholic? Although you already know, it is often on a subconscious level. You may not be aware yet on a conscious level. You may need some prodding.

Let's start with the conventional criteria. Answer yes or no to the following:

DO YOU DRINK EVERY DAY?

Consuming alcohol every day produces brain chemical changes that create a physiological addiction. Even if you don't feel addicted or notice a psychological addiction, there are changes in your body chemistry that now require the presence of alcohol and, with time, will cause other adverse chemical changes when alcohol is withdrawn. When exposed to alcohol, some of the neurotransmitters in the brain's nerve cells rapidly acquire the need for alcohol to function, and they malfunction when it is withdrawn. Of course, the severe form of this is DTs, but, even with continuous moderate alcohol consumption, there are subtle unpleasant biochemical and physiological changes when alcohol is withdrawn. Perhaps it is just an uneasiness or mild depression when you skip a day of drinking. So consciously or not, you learn not to miss a day. You're addicted.

HAVE YOU LOST A JOB BECAUSE OF DRINKING?

This is one of the classic definitions of alcoholism and one of the most valid for the obvious abuser. But short of being terminated, there are more subtle signs in the workplace of an excessive fondness for drink that are suggestive of a growing problem. Maybe it's missing work or chronic tardiness because you were hung over from a night of drinking. Perhaps it is poor job performance, anger, or quarrelsome behavior brought on by the drinking. These signs are clearly identifiable, and few would argue they are the results of an alcohol problem. But for every drinker who loses his job or struggles on with barely tolerable evaluations because of these obvious problems, there are ten workplace HFAs who chronically underperform at work because of alcohol. They accomplish little after noon because of their two-drink lunches causing drowsiness during the second half of the day. They get no take-home work done because they are worthless once they start drinking in the evening.

In the liberated days of the sixties, when the baby boomers experimented with drugs, much was made of the amotivational syndrome caused by chronic marijuana use. The old aphorism "going to pot" was coined a half century before sophisticated psychological tests defined the problem. Alcohol has the same effect on many people, creating a personal inertia that slows their careers, financial growth, and personal development. When one has a blood alcohol level of 0.1 percent every night, it's hard to get much done.

HAVE YOU ENDED A RELATIONSHIP BECAUSE OF DRINKING?

Divorce or its equivalent is one of the most common occurrences in an alcoholic's life. The alcoholic creates so many impassable roadblocks in the relationship that it turns into a nightmare for the nonalcoholic partner. Whether it is economic insecurity from being fired for drinking on the job, verbal or physical abuse, social embarrassment, or just the growing realization that alcohol is more important than the relationship, the nonalcoholic spouse or partner endures a series of hellish experiences before finally giving up. Oftentimes, the resultant breakup causes the alcoholic to spin further out of control.

But just as there are untold thousands of workplace alcoholics whose behavior never reaches the threshold for termination, there are millions of men and women who struggle in silence with partners who are chronically intoxicated, rude, and deprecating and make the lives of their significant others barely tolerable. At a party, Molly averts her eyes when Larry spills his wine or makes a rude remark. But she is always there to drive him home, enabling him to continue his alcoholism. Molly's insecurity keeps her there. A relationship with a drunk is better than no relationship at all. Does this sound familiar? Does alcohol dominate your relationship?

HAVE YOU BEEN ARRESTED FOR DRUNK DRIVING?

For many alcoholics, this is the wake-up call that they have lost touch with the seriousness of their drinking. It is public humiliation, and it is often the jolt they need to realize that their life is in a downward spiral. Many seek help and find it. Others, still deep in denial, just curse their bad luck at getting caught, hire an attorney who is expert at damage control, and go on with their intoxicated lives. Alcoholics are conditioned to blame their problems on other people or fate. Rarely do they take responsibility.

Wisely, many states require the person cited for DUI to take a class or enroll in an alcohol rehab program. Another excellent idea would be to sentence the convicted DUI to forty hours of volunteer work at the local alcohol detox unit. For many early-stage alcoholics, a close-up look at where they are heading is shocking enough to bring about long-term change. Drunk drivers are frequently sentenced to hours of community service, but, too often, they can pick and choose their assignment, and there is no learning or behavior modification that results. I volunteer with the local state park maintaining trails. At a recent work project, we had two convicted DUIs fulfilling their community service requirement. One was so hung over that he was worthless; the other drove to the eight o'clock project reeking of booze. There was no real supervision or any negative consequences for continued alcoholic behavior.

For every convicted drunk driver, there are a multitude of social drinkers who regularly drive home from parties with blood alcohol levels greater than 0.08 percent, the legal limit in most states. Are you one of them? The fact we try to get away with it is good evidence that alcohol impairs judgment. Driving under the influence also erodes morality. We know it is wrong, but do it anyway. We are on the slippery slope of alcoholism, explaining away verbal or physical abuse or adultery, behaviors we disparage when sober. It is such a subtle line that we don't realize we have crossed it. And alcohol facilitated our crossing.

ARE YOU RESTLESS AND ILL AT EASE WHEN NOT DRINKING?

The anxiety many alcoholics experience when sober is a combination of feeling socially ill at ease without some alcohol in their bloodstream and actual physiological withdrawal caused by malfunctioning neurons in the brain that have become dependent on the presence of alcohol to work correctly. The alcoholic enters a social gathering looking for the bar. Once it is located, he immediately has two drinks. He wants a quick effect, and one is not enough. If he is unlucky enough to be invited to a Baptist wedding with the reception in the social hall of the church, precluding alcohol, he doesn't stay long. Or he has a couple drinks before the wedding and a flask to keep the buzz going at the reception. In my drinking days, I attended a men's retreat at the Mission San Antonio. We were in prayer and discussion groups all day. At dinner, I was surprised I felt an almost desperate desire for a beer. As we sat down to eat, I noticed a bottle of jug wine on the table. I used to collect good wine, but I had no appetite for bulk wine. Despite that, I had several glasses to satisfy my craving. I just wanted the alcohol, and it did make me feel better, although I was disgusted with myself for so desperately needing those drinks. It was ten years before I could finally summon the personal and spiritual strength to banish alcohol from my life.

HAVE YOU HAD BLACKOUTS AFTER DRINKING?

A young man in my fraternity literally became psychotic when he was drunk. Chris Putnam was six-foot-two and two hundred and twenty pounds without an ounce of fat, and he had been recruited to play center for our top-rated college football team. He was in my pledge class in the fraternity, and it was our responsibility to keep him in check when he drank. It was an impossible job. After a number of beers, Chris would become a one-man wrecking crew, throwing chairs through windows, putting his fist through walls, and wrestling with anyone he could get his hands on. It was terrifying to see him on the rampage. Several of the bigger and more sober brothers frequently knocked Chris unconscious just to end the siege.

The next morning, Chris was a lamb, and he had no recollection of the night before. Having never been so drunk that I couldn't remember my actions, I thought he was copping out. He wasn't. I've since learned that many young men and women experience blackouts when they drink heavily. The conventional wisdom is that such episodes are not a sign of serious alcoholism and young people grow out of these phases. This is wrong thinking. If a person has a seizure, we put him on medication to prevent future seizures, and we rescind his driver's license to prevent injury to himself or others. Why should we be more lenient with the alcoholic who has blackouts? Anyone who gets drunk and violent and can't remember the episode should consider his drinking life threatening and seek help immediately.

If you answered yes to one or more of the previous questions, you are an alcoholic. You are not alone. Between 15 and 30 percent of men and 10 to 15 percent of women will answer yes to one of the above accepted criteria for alcoholism. There are, however, more subtle indications of a growing problem. Answer yes or no to the following:

CAN YOU HAVE JUST ONE DRINK?

Or does one drink make you feel just a tiny bit mellow but you know you'd feel even better if you had another? Or maybe two? The HFA is in search of that little buzz, and one drink doesn't get him there. If you drink looking for a feeling, you are a problem drinker.

DO YOU DRINK ALONE?

If you drink alone, perhaps you are drinking to relax after a hard day at work. While there's nothing wrong with that per se, it means you have chosen a chemical form of relaxation that is addictive. You are using alcohol like a drug, tranquilizer, or antianxiety drug. Why not take a Valium or smoke a joint? Anyway you look at it, it's a drug addiction. You have a problem.

DO YOU CRAVE A DRINK?

Does your mouth water at the thought of that first beer? Does your hand tremble as you unscrew the cap, waiting for the ice-cold effervescence? You are conditioned, like Pavlov's dogs. They were reacting to a ringing bell, and you're reacting to the concrete representation of a substance that's going to make you feel good. Like a heroin addict who begins to sweat when he heats the mixture in a spoon, your mind and body are anticipating the high. You are kidding yourself if you think it's just a social habit. It's a drug habit.

DO YOU DRINK DURING THE DAY?

I spent a summer watching a hard-core alcoholic in action. He had his first beer between nine and ten in the morning. He still had a significant level of alcohol in his bloodstream from the night before. As it dropped, all the brain chemicals that are dependent on a certain blood concentration of alcohol began to malfunction, and Larry became restless and cranky. But after the first couple of beers, he visibly relaxed. From that point on, he drank steadily throughout the day and night. If you drink during the day, you may be responding to subtle physiological symptoms that are being communicated from your body. Symptoms that are saying, "I'll feel much better if I have a couple of beers." So you do. And you feel better. Unfortunately, you will have to continue to drink during the remainder of your waking hours, or you will revert to that edgy feeling. If this is you, you need to stop.

DO YOU DRIVE DRUNK?

Do you drive after drinking more than three or four ounces of alcohol within several hours? The California Highway Patrol estimates that, on major urban freeways and road systems after dark, 5 percent of all drivers on the road are legally drunk. Legally drunk is a blood alcohol level of 0.08 percent. For my height and weight (six-foot-one and one hundred and eighty pounds), that's three beers. A beer is an ounce of alcohol. Your liver can metabolize alcohol to acetaldehyde at a rate of one ounce per hour. If you drink more than that, your blood alcohol level climbs until you stop or pass out.

Driving drunk is a learned skill. It is amazing how the nervous system can adjust to intoxication. Many people who drink a lot can drive reasonably well when they can barely stand, with a blood alcohol level of 0.2 percent, for example. And so they do it. Have you?

You avoid freeways and drive surface streets where there is less scrutiny. You deliberately go the speed limit or slightly slower so as not to attract attention. But driving too slowly or speeding will draw equal attention. If you add just the least little weave, you may be blowing into a breathalyzer. Ironically, good drunk drivers are usually excellent sober drivers and, as a result, rarely get caught. But every now and then, they slip up. A good friend was pulled over for a burned-out taillight, not for impaired driving, but the CHP immediately recognized he'd been drinking. He failed a field sobriety test and a breathalyzer, as his blood alcohol level was 0.18 percent. He spent a night in jail and lost his license for six months.

Another friend used to joke he was a better driver drunk than most other people were sober, remarking elderly drivers have bad eyesight and slow reaction times and are dangerously timid or slow. What he is not acknowledging is that his reaction time in an emergency is three or four times longer drunk than it is sober. The ability to brake in a timely manner, avoid obstacles on the road, and avoid other vehicles is dangerously altered. He is a menace to himself and those in his vehicle and a threat to everyone around him. But being self-absorbed is a common trait of an alcoholic, so rarely do the safety or rights of other individuals enter into his thinking. He is also ignoring the fact that driving while intoxicated is against the law. Eleven thousand alcohol related highway fatalities occur each year, equaling nearly a quarter of the deaths resulting from the Vietnam War (Vietnam War Casualties). When eight of our servicemen die in a training exercise, the entire nation mourns. But sixty deaths on the highway occur every day in this country. In 50 percent of those deaths, alcohol has played a role. So a wounded nation, seeking to protect itself, set an arbitrary and low limit of 0.08 percent as legally drunk. If you are caught, you will be busted. There is a zero-tolerance rule in the evaluation of highway drunkenness. And that is as it should be.

DO YOU SAY THINGS WHEN YOU ARE DRINKING THAT YOU LATER REGRET?

Alcohol loosens tongues. We all have many conversations going on in our minds at any given time. There is the reality conversation, taking in the scene around us, evaluating it, and reacting. But simultaneously, we have tangential thoughts—some critical, some angry, and some frankly paranoid—vying for our attention. We have all had thoughts we were ashamed of, which we know are untrue. When we are sober, we keep these thoughts in check. When we're drunk, they often just come out:

You can only hope the wounds are not fatal to one you love or a relationship you cherish. So you bind the wounds, ask for forgiveness, and let healing occur. But you need to be aware that alcohol can amplify any anger in you, and it will hurt you and the ones you love. It's not worth the buzz to lose control this way.

DO YOU CONCEAL THE AMOUNT YOU DRINK FROM YOUR FRIENDS OR SIGNIFICANT OTHER?

One excellent strategy to force a person to recognize he has a significant problem with alcohol is to count the number of ounces of alcohol he consumes. Confronted with the actual volume of intoxicant, many heavy drinkers are unable to deny they have a problem.

The drinker in denial, however, goes to great lengths to conceal the actual amount he is drinking. If he drinks hard liquor, he may have a secret stash from which he refills the bottle in the cupboard so it is not apparent how much he really consumes. The wine drinker may have two or three bottles in the fridge and tipples from all of them so the amount consumed is not readily apparent. Beer drinkers have a spare six-pack or two in the cupboard and replace each one as it is drunk so the fridge always looks full. Having several different brands on hand also helps to confuse the issue. If you conduct this kind of alcoholic sleight of hand, you have a problem.

DO YOU USE MINTS OR MOUTHWASH TO COVER THE SMELL OF ALCOHOL ON YOUR BREATH?

Doubtless because I have had my own issues with alcohol, I am extremely aware of what I sense to be problems in others. HFAs are usually pretty cagey though, and some are paranoid or ashamed enough to want to hide the problem from others. Like some smokers who use mouthwash to hide the smoke on their breath, many drinkers are acutely aware that alcohol is readily detectable on the breath. They have breath mints in their pocket or purse or carry one of those little spray bottles of mouthwash in the car or on their person. This is premeditation. It means they drink regularly and seek to cover it up, a sign of a serious problem. Is this you?

ARE YOU TIRED OF BEING A SLAVE TO ALCOHOL?

Reread the preceding questions, and answer yes or no to each one. Be honest with yourself. If you have one question answered affirmatively, you have a drinking problem, and you are heading for a bigger one in the future. It is time to admit it and look for help.

45

HOW I GOT SOBER

Many of my friends and a few readers refuse to believe I am really an alcoholic. In recent years, none had ever seen me obviously drunk. They claim the quantities I drank and the frequency of my drinking would never qualify me as a drunk. They cling to the notion that an alcoholic has to live in a constant state of drunkenness, get involved in bar brawls, accumulate DUIs, and lose his job, spouse, and home. Right in front of their noses are family members and coworkers who are stealth drinkers like I was, drinking steadily day in and day out, uncomfortable as heck at a wedding or party where alcohol is not served, and progressively moving toward higher consumption and greater need. Or perhaps my story makes them uncomfortable because it hits too close to home and they are unwilling to admit they might have a problem.

So let's look at the facts:

- I drank nearly every day, almost exclusively beer, because, with beer, I could easily modulate my level of intoxication. I kept myself in that sweet spot of feel good and no worries, somewhere between no effect at all and getting sloppy. I could drink beer all afternoon and evening and maintain the perfect level. At least, that's how it worked in the early days. But, in reality, I used alcohol as a drug, no different than if I were taking Valium or OxyContin.
- My drinking was progressive. After brief failed interludes of abstention, I couldn't return to social drinking of one or two beers. Within a week, I'd be back at the

high-volume, high-frequency drinking that preceded the break. Oftentimes, there was a step up to a higher volume.
- I didn't have control over my drinking. Once I started, I drank until I reached my sweet spot, whatever that took. Just because I didn't drink myself unconscious doesn't mean I didn't have a problem.
- Alcohol changed my personality. I became critical, argumentative, cynical, and sullen. I could feel it happening after the first beer. I drank in search of my pleasure place, but, more and more often, I didn't get there. Instead, I'd go to the dark side. I knew something was wrong, but I wasn't sure what. I believe much of it was depression, but I was unable to label it at the time.
- I couldn't quit. I hated the way alcohol made me feel. I hated the nightly failure as I broke my daily vow and took the first drink. I felt so humiliated, so powerless, and so ashamed. But I couldn't help myself. I can understand why a hopeless alcoholic could choose suicide. There is no other way out.

Does this description sound like a social drinker? Does it sound like a normal person who periodically drinks too much? Anyone who cannot see the problem I have may have one of his own.

True alcoholics come in all sizes, shapes, and colors. They have bottoms in the depths of hell or just off the bell-shaped curve of normal drinking. I have a friend who quit drinking because he missed a single day of work with a hangover. He has over fifty years of sobriety and helped countless men get sober. Conventional wisdom would never label him an alcoholic, but it is clear he is one when you hear his story and understand the problem. He just had the incredible good fortune to realize where the road was leading before it led him off the cliff. Many of us who have found sobriety and serenity wonder why we are so fortunate when so many others still suffer. There is not an easy answer. We just call it grace, and we are humbly grateful.

It didn't just happen. I didn't wake up on Ash Wednesday 2001 and miraculously stop drinking. There had been countless failed attempts previously, but this time was different. This time, after my abject humiliation at the New Year's Eve party, I finally admitted I was powerless to get sober on my own, yet I wanted sobriety more than anything else in the world. So I kneeled down and admitted to my higher power that I was helpless and asked Him to take charge of my life. I surrendered. It was the first time in my life that I completely surrendered my ego, my self-centered control of everything around me. It wasn't just words. It was true and absolute surrender. The burden was no longer mine alone. Suddenly, the strength was there.

They say there are no atheists in foxholes in the heat of battle. The same could be said of men and women who have worked the first three of the twelve steps of AA. Some call it God, some call it their higher power, and some call it the group conscience. It doesn't seem to matter as long as the surrender is genuine. The miracle that happens, the grace that is conferred, is just as genuine.

Once I had been gifted with the critical foundation of spiritual strength, I still had to deal with the physical problems that would be obstacles to continuing sobriety. I knew I would not succeed unless I could keep myself from lifting an ice-cold beer to my lips. That was the challenge. I had some insights from years of drinking and failed attempts to quit. I knew I craved the high I got with alcohol, but I also realized that part of the relief I felt when I drank was the rapid correction of a low blood sugar. Remember, ethanol functions as a two-carbon sugar. It is absorbed right through the mucosae of the mouth, esophagus, stomach, and intestine. It doesn't need to be transported into the intestine or digested. It's instantaneous. So part of the physical benefit of drinking, say at the end of a long workday, was getting my blood sugar up where I felt normal. The first physical change I had to make was to find something else to take its place. Many years before, I had discovered I could successfully diet by eating carrots when I felt hungry. Because I have a huge bag of carrots in the barn to provide treats for the horses, it seemed like the first thing to try. I stopped making my nightly swing by the liquor store for a six-pack and stuck a big carrot in my mouth as soon as I reached the barn. Within a few minutes, the emptiness in my stomach disappeared. Over time and out of necessity, I tried other foods to see if they could cut the craving. A glass of milk, some cheese, and eating an energy bar, all worked very well.

Over the past twenty-two years, I have learned to carry an energy bar in my briefcase, and I have cheese in the fridge at the office. I never let my blood sugar get too low, which has greatly diminished the craving for alcohol. I also have learned that, if I am sober, I am much less likely to experience hypoglycemia. Alcohol prevents the liver from storing glycogen (long chains of glucose), which can be released to buffer an episode of hypoglycemia. Additionally, my knowledge of diminishing cravings really helped my abstinence. I knew that, if I could make it a week or two without drinking, I would have a good chance of finally quitting.

But, once sober, I began to see that was not enough. I needed to know what it was that made me need to drink, get drunk, and be addicted. One of my mentors, Bud Beecher, loaned me *Adult Children of Alcoholics* by Timmen Cermak, MD. There, I read a psychological portrait of myself, and so many things made sense. It is beyond the scope of this book to explore the many dynamics of the ACA, but I am gradually coming to grips with the way I was raised and the profound effect it continues to have on me.

I did not gain sobriety as a member of AA, but I have since joined and found a wonderful group of men with whom I meet regularly. I would have never envisioned myself in AA, but I love it. I appreciate the fellowship of so many remarkable men with decades of sobriety. Some of these wise, old owls have profound insights into alcoholism and a venerable sense of calm contentedness that is a cherished goal for my life. Almost every week, there is someone with less than thirty days of sobriety or someone who has been out and is trying to get back in. Seeing those struggling souls, I silently thank God for his gift of my sobriety.

AA advocates a twelve-step program that has the potential to transform one's life. It can be found in the appendix of this book. The twelve steps are the blueprint for a spiritual awakening from which anyone, sober or not, could benefit. I have progressed to the difficult steps, four through nine. Admitting all my wrongs to another person, revealing the dark episodes of my drunken past, and then making amends, where possible, is a challenge. I am sure that completing the steps will be as hard as getting sober. But contentment and inner peace will be the reward.

In AA, it is said you have to change everything about your life. That's not always true. When you get sober, everything will change around you, as it did for me. I've been married for thirty-five years, and my wife likes me much better sober. She never drank much and drinks even less now, and she is very supportive of my mission to wake up as many people as possible to the disaster alcohol can create for them. The most significant change is that many of my old friends have drifted away. Most of them drink, some a lot. My sobriety is threatening to them, so they prefer not to have me at their parties. That's okay with me. I miss them and their friendships, but at least two have gotten sober since I did, and now we have even more in common.

I lost my dad six years ago to gastric carcinoma, a cancer known to be caused by alcohol and tobacco, both of which he abused. He was a dear, sweet man whom I loved unreservedly, but his high-functioning alcoholism of five decades deteriorated in the last fifteen years of his life. White wine and vodka salved the aches, pains, and grief of aging. He knew I was sober, but he didn't really know how I felt about his drinking. It was just one more in a multitude of denials.

My mother lives in a quiet senior residence. She drinks a lot less than she did when Dad was alive. Like him, she is not consciously aware that their lives were dominated by drinking or how it affected my siblings and me.

Both my sisters drink, but not to excess. They are aware of our parents' problem, but they don't yet understand the profound ways such an upbringing has affected them. They both understand and support my recovery, for which I am grateful.

The most profound change is my delight at learning who I am sober and discovering I genuinely love the person I am becoming. If you really work the steps of AA, you become a disarmingly honest person. It is so freeing to be honest and to learn to admit mistakes without feeling less worthy of love because of it. Thomas Merton speaks of the true self. I am becoming my true self. There is a sense of awe and gratitude in that. I can experience peace and happiness I didn't think possible and the hole in my soul is filled with a fire that, I pray, will light the darkness for brothers and sisters who suffer as I did.

THE SOBERING TRUTH

46

INFORMED CONSENT

As a physician, a large proportion of what I do is educating and informing patients. When I see a patient, my first task is to make a diagnosis. No treatment is possible without an accurate diagnosis. In arriving there, it is often necessary to perform certain tests like biopsies, blood tests, and other sophisticated procedures. An important part of my job is informing patients of the possible negative consequences of these investigations. Similarly, once I have arrived at a diagnosis, I will recommend one or more possible treatments. There may be topical creams to control the problem. Perhaps an oral medication is the most efficacious. There are times when a laser procedure is the best option. In the case of cancer, perhaps surgery or even radiation is the most appropriate.

At every step along the way, it is my job to educate and inform the patient as to what the possible consequences of the testing or treatment may be. This is a time-consuming and difficult task, but an extremely important one. Patients need to be able to make educated choices and appreciate, in terms they can understand, the pros and cons of all their diagnostic and therapeutic options.

In a society in which the medical-legal ramifications of any drug therapy or procedure may result in huge liability payouts, it is somewhat laughable the length that drug manufacturers and physicians go to adequately present their possible negative effects. If you consider the ultimate worst-case scenario, the possibility of life-altering changes and even death have to be included in almost every informed consent. In the double-speak world, we sometimes don't talk about a patient's death. We call it a negative patient outcome. I am treating a young and knowledgeable physician with a potentially hazardous drug that requires a signed informed consent before therapy. When he got done reading it, he signed it, handed it back to me, and said, "If patients really read and understand these things, it is remarkable that any one would take this drug."

It is part of our optimistic nature that we can't accept that any of those bad things are going to happen to us. But we still need to know that the possibility exists.

So it is with alcohol. We drink it and enjoy the effect it has, but we may not know all the really negative consequences of our drinking. Even in an age when denial is the most prevalent emotion, allowing some incredibly dangerous behaviors, perhaps we should enumerate the possible results of drinking. Unlike the rare side effects of some of the medications we prescribe, many of these consequences will occur to the person who drinks habitually. We all need to know these things, especially young people who are just being introduced to drinking and still have an objective viewpoint. Looking back, when I was a teenager, I wish I had a clear idea where drinking might take me. I wish I had read a book like this and had a chance to realize what I was doing to my body and mind.

For many young people, reading this will not prevent them from drinking. The pressure to conform and power of the peer group is too strong. But for some, this catalog of alcohol's woes will open their eyes. It is for them that this chapter and this book were written.

A detailed explanation of each of these problems can be found within the pages of this book. The Informed Consent for the Consumption of Alcohol follows. If you would like to use it for a discussion group, copies can be downloaded from our website at www.soberingtruth.com.

INFORMED CONSENT

THE SOBERING TRUTH

INFORMED CONSENT FOR THE CONSUMPTION OF ALCOHOL

DATE:_____

I, _____, have been thoroughly informed of the risks of drinking alcohol. Specifically, I have been informed of the following (initial each statement):

_____ Alcohol can be addictive.

_____ Alcohol is a poison.

_____ Alcohol can cause cancer of the mouth, throat, esophagus, stomach, colon, pancreas, liver, and prostate.

_____ If I already have had cancer, alcohol can allow it to spread throughout my body.

_____ Alcohol can cause osteoporosis (weakening of my bones).

_____ Alcohol can make my allergies worse.

_____ Alcohol can cause insomnia (sleeplessness).

_____ Alcohol can cause severe heartburn or gastroesophageal reflux disease (GERD)

_____ Alcohol can weaken my immune system.

_____ Alcohol can cause hepatitis, progressing to cirrhosis.

_____ Alcohol can cause pancreatitis.

_____ Alcohol can weaken my heart.

_____ Alcohol can cause obesity.

_____ Alcohol can cause diabetes.

_____ Alcohol can cause hypoglycemia (low blood sugar).

_____ Alcohol can cause memory loss and dementia.

_____ Alcohol can cause neuropathy (a painful burning of the hands and feet).

INFORMED CONSENT

_____ Even small amounts of alcohol can cause birth defects.

_____ Alcohol can increase my risk of breast cancer six times the national average (women only)

_____ Alcohol can cause aggressive behavior.

_____ Alcohol can lead to unwanted sexual encounters.

_____ Alcohol can lead to sexually transmitted diseases.

_____ Alcohol can lead to unplanned pregnancies.

_____ Alcohol can cause severe depression.

_____ Alcohol can cause suicide.

_____ Alcohol can lead to other dangerous addictions.

_____ I understand that alcohol can get me arrested.

_____ I understand that alcohol is a factor in 32% of fatal highway accidents.

_____ I understand that alcohol is a factor in 48% of all homicides.

_____ I understand that alcohol is a factor in 55% of all spousal abuse.

I certify that I am of sound mind and body and have made the decision to drink alcohol, having understood all the possible consequences and considered the risks. I make this decision of my own accord and will hold no one else responsible. I am not giving in to peer pressure from my friends just because I want to be accepted as one of the group. I hold harmless the manufacturers and marketers of alcohol as I feel I have been adequately informed of the physical and psychological risks of drinking alcohol.

Signed:_____ Date:_____

WORKS CITED

Alcoholics Anonymous. 4th ed.
New York: Alcoholics Anonymous World Services, 2001.

Anon. University of Pittsburgh School of Medicine.
"Student Affairs Handbook, 2005."
http://www.medschool.pitt. edu/studentaffairs/alcohol.html.

Anon. Vietnam War Casualties. 2003.
http://www.vietnamwarinfo/casualties.

CDC Fact Book 2001-2002. www.cdc.gov/ncipc/fact_book_ different.htm.

Children of Alcoholics Foundation, Inc. "Collaboration, Coordination, and Cooperation: Helping Children Affected by Parental Addiction and Family Violence", New York, 1996.

Enzinger, C. et al. Risk factors for progression of brain atrophy in aging: Six-year follow-up of normal subjects. Neurology 64: 1704–1706.

Jefferis, B.J. et al. Adolescent drinking level and adult binge drinking in a national birth cohort. *Addiction* 100: 543–549.

Miller, J.W. et al. Prevalence of adult binge drinking: A comparison of two national surveys.
American Journal of Preventive Medicine 27(3): 197–204.

Morbidity and Mortality Weekly Report (MMWR). 53(22): 471–474.

Morbidity and Mortality Weekly Report (MMWR). 54: 377–380.

Nadeau, Remi. *Ft. Laramie and the Sioux.*
Santa Barbara: Crest Publishers 1997, pp 34 and 41.

Rumbaugh, C. L. et al. *Investigative Radiology* 11: 282–294.

Sesso, HD er al. Int J Epidemiol 2001 Aug 30 (4) 749-55.

Wrensch, M et al. *Breast Cancer Research* 5(4) R 88-102. EPub 2003 April 29.

APPENDIX ONE

ALCOHOL AND CANCER

Homann, N. Alcohol's breakdown product acetaldehyde is toxic, mutagenic, and carcinogenic. *Addict Biol* 6(4): 309–323.

Key, T.J. Alcohol increases risk of breast cancer. *Lancet Oncol* 2(3): 133–140.

Li, D. Alcohol may promote pancreatic cancer by increasing K-ras mutation. *Cancer J* 7(4): 259–265.

Mufti, S.J. Alcohol promotes cancer of the gastrointestinal tract. *Cancer Detect Prev* 22(3): 195–203.

Noda, T. Alcoholics have higher mortality rates from all cancers. *Psychiatry Clin Neurosci* 55(5): 466–472.

Novak, R.F. Alcohol increases CYP2E1 variant of cytochrome P450, which may promote cancer development. *Arch Pharm Res* 23(4): 267–282.

Schottenfeld, D. Alcohol is an important factor in causing liver cancer. *Cancer* 43(5 suppl): 1962–1966.

Sesso, H.D. et al. 2001. Alcohol consumption and risk of prostate cancer: The Harvard alumni health study. *Int J Epidemiology* 30(4): 749–755.

Thomas, D.B. Alcohol and tobacco account for 80 percent of cancer of the mouth, pharynx, larynx, and esophagus in the United States. *Environ Health Perspect* 103(Suppl 8): 153–160.

Thun, M.J. Alcohol increases death rate from breast cancer by 30 percent. *N Engl J Med* 337(24): 1705–1714.

Wrensch, M. Alcohol may be partially responsible for higher rates of breast cancer in Marin County, California, than elsewhere. *Breast Cancer Res* 5(4): R88–R102.

Wu, W.J. Alcohol decreases host resistance to spread of melanoma. *Int J Cancer* 82(6): 886–892.

ALCOHOL AND THE HEART
Li, Y. et al. 2009. *Eur J Cancer* 45(5): 843–850.

ALCOHOL AND HYPERTENSION
Sesso, H.D. et al. 2008. *Hypertension* 51(4): 1080–1087.

ALCOHOL AND OSTEOPOROSIS
Faine, M.P. Alcohol increases urinary loss of calcium.
J Prosthet Dent 73(1): 65–72.

Laitinen, K. Increased urinary excretion of calcium and decreased serum calcium are noted eight hours after alcohol intake.
N Engl J Med 324(11): 721–727.

Nishiguchi, S. Alcohol decreases bone mineral density, greater in females than in males. *J Bone Miner Metab* 18(6): 317–320.

Ringe, J.D. Alcohol is second most important risk factor in osteoporosis in men. *Dtsch Med Wochenschr* 119(27): 943–947.

Zima, T. Alcohol causes decreased parathyroid hormone, thus lowering calcium. *Sb Lek* 94(4): 303–309.

ALCOHOL AND ENCEPHALOPATHY
Enzinger, C. et al. 2005. Risk factors for progression of brain atrophy in aging: Six-year follow-up of normal subjects. *Neurology* 64: 1704–1706.

ALCOHOL AND IMMUNITY
Chang, M.P. Alcohol suppresses T lymphocyte proliferation.
Int J Immunopharmacol 14(4): 707–719.

Gonzalez-Quintana, A. 2002. Alcohol increases IGE levels.
Alcohol Clin Exp Rev 26: 60–64.

Grossman, C.J. Alcohol decreases maturation of thymic T cells.
Int J Immunopharmacol 10(2): 187–195.

Na, H. R. Alcohol suppresses cell-mediated immunity.
Alcohol Clin Exp Rev 21(7): 1179–1185.

Wang, Y. Vit E blocks alcohol-induced immune suppression.
Alcohol Clin Exp Rev 18(2): 355–362.

Wu, W.J. Alcohol decreases natural killer T cells.
Int J Cancer 82(6): 886–892.

ALCOHOL AND GASTROESOPHAGEAL REÀUX DISEASE (GERD)

Bujanda, L. Alcohol decreases force of contraction of esophageal muscle and weakens sphincter while increasing stomach acid production.
Am J Gastroenterol 95(12): 3374–3382.

Choy, D. Gastroesophageal reflux may cause asthma by stimulating the vagus nerve, and asthma may cause GERD by changing esophageal dynamics via altered diaphragmatic movement.
Respirology 2(3): 163–168.

Kaufman, S.E. Alcohol causes GERD. *Gut* 19(4): 336–338.

Vitale, J.C. Alcohol significantly increases the acidity of the distal esophagus by permitting increased reflux of stomach acid.
JAMA 258(15): 2077–2079.

FETAL ALCOHOL SYNDROME

Burd, L. et al. 2007. *Cong Heart Dis* 2(4): 2508. Calhoun, F. 2007. *Neuro Sci Biobehav Rev* 31(2): 168–171. Camarillo, C. et al. 2008. *Gene Expr* 14(3): 159–171. Chee, J. 2007. *Acta Neuropathology* 113(6): 659–673. Fryer, S.L. 2007. *Pediatrics* 119(3): 733–741. Gemma, S. 2006. *Ann Ist Super Sanita* 42(1): 8–16. Green, F.F. et al. 2007. *Am J Obstet Gynecol* 197(1): 12–25.

Guizzeti, M. et al. 2007. *Hema Exp Toxical* 26(4): 355–360.

Gundogan, F. et al. 2008. *Placenta* 29(2): 148–157.

Ieraci, A. 2007. *Neurobiol Dis* (3): 597–605.

J et al. 2008. *Neuroendocrine* 20(4): 470–488.

Jiang, Q. 2007. *Alcohol* 42(4): 285–290.

Koditowakko, P.W. 2007. *Neurosci Biobehavior Rev* 31(2): 192–201.

Li, Y.X. 2007. *Lab Invest* (3): 231–240. Mayoch, D.E. 2007. *J Appl Physiol* 102(3): 972–977. McGee, C.L. 2008. *Am J Drug Alcohol Abuse* 34(4): 423–431.

Merrick, J. 2006. *Minerva Pediatrics* 58(3): 211–218.

Miller, M.W. et al. 2006. *Alcohol Clin Exp Res* 30(9): 1466–1469.

Northwest Portland area maternal child health newsletter. *Pediatrics* 106(2): 358–360.

Pragst F. et al. 2008. *Ther Drug Monitor* 30(2): 255–263 [4].

Rao V. et al. 2007. **Alcohol** 41(6) 433–439.

Rasmussen, C. et al. 2006. *Child Neuropsychology* 12(6): 453–468.

Servais, L. 2007. *Proc Nat Acad Sci USA* 104 (23) : 9858–9863.

Shankar, K. et al. 2006. *Exp Biol Med (Maywood)*(8): 1379–1397.

Spohr, H.L. 2007. *J Pediatc* 150(2): 175–179.

Vaglenova, J. et al. 2008. *Neuropsycho pharmacology* 33(5): 107–183.

Yelim, R. 2007. *Differentiation* 75(5): 393–403.

APPENDIX TWO

THE TWELVE STEPS OF ALCOHOLICS ANONYMOUS

STEP 1 We admitted we were powerless over alcohol—that our lives had become unmanageable.

STEP 2 Came to believe that a power greater than ourselves could restore us to sanity.

STEP 3 Made a decision to turn our will and our lives over to the care of God as we understood Him.

STEP 4 Made a searching and fearless moral inventory of ourselves.

STEP 5 Admitted to God, to ourselves, and to another human being the exact nature of our wrongs.

STEP 6 Were entirely ready to have God remove all these defects of character.

STEP 7 Humbly asked Him to remove our shortcomings.

STEP 8 Made a list of all persons we had harmed, and became willing to make amends to them all.

STEP 9 Made direct amends to such people wherever possible, except when to do so would injure them or others.

STEP 10 Continued to take personal inventory and when we were wrong promptly admitted it.

STEP 11 Sought through prayer and meditation to improve our conscious contact with God, as we understood him, praying only for knowledge of his will for us and the power to carry that out.

STEP 12 Having had a spiritual awakening as a result of these steps, we tried to carry this message to alcoholics and to practice these principles in all our affairs.

THE SOBERING TRUTH

www.ingramcontent.com/pod-product-compliance
Lightning Source LLC
Chambersburg PA
CBHW060455030426
42337CB00015B/1596